# OVERCOME WHAT YOUR BRAIN CANNOT

*Retrain your brain to respond the way it did prior to experiencing illness, physical trauma, or emotional injury including stroke, chronic pain, fibromyalgia, and neuropathy.*

## DR. RICHARD HERMAN

Contact information:

Dr. Richard Herman

Drrichardherman@gmail.com

# TABLE OF CONTENTS:

**Introduction**        p.1

Chapter 1:   **A New Understanding**        p.5

Chapter 2:   **Neuroreactive Injury Formation**        p.15

Chapter 3:   **Exploring Treatments That Can Help You Get Better**        p.23

Chapter 4:   **Overcoming The Way Others View Your Chronic Nonstructural Injury**        p.47

## Part Two

*Applying A Neuroreactive Approach To Overcome A Brain That Prevents Itself From Recovering*

Chapter 5:   **The Brain That Refused To Overcome Acute and Chronic Illness**        p.57

Chapter 6:   **The Diabetic Brain**        p.67

Chapter 7:   **The Brain That Refused To Heal Itself After A Stroke**        p.81

Chapter 8:   **The Brain That Refused To Allow Itself To Recover From Physical Injury**        p.91

Chapter 9:  **The Brain That Allowed Itself**          p.109
            **To Recover From A Surgery**
            **Before  It Underwent The Procedure**

Chapter 10: **The Brain That Avoided The Need**        p.125
            **For Anesthesia During Surgery**

Chapter 11: **The Brain That Refused To Allow Itself** p.135
            **To Overcome Emotional Issues And**
            **Interactive Trauma**

Chapter 12: **The Brain That Refused To**              p.153
            **Allow Itself To Remember Any**
            **Memories Of The Past**

Chapter 13: **The Brain That Refused To Allow**        p.161
            **The Body To Lose Weight**

Chapter 14: **The Brain That Refused To Allow**        p.175
            **Itself To Go To The Dentist**

Chapter 15: **Legal Implications That May Result**     p.181
            **From A Brain That Refuses To Allow**
            **Itself To Get Better**

Chapter 16: **The Brain That Allowed Itself To Heal**  p.187
            **By Responding To Placebos**

            **Index:**                                 p.199

# INTRODUCTION

The inspiration for this book is a direct result of the time and ongoing research that has been thrust on me. It was not the path that I had envisioned that I would lead. My journey started out with the birth of my son, Joshua. Over the first two years of his life, it became apparent that he was not meeting the developmental milestones that all the other kids his age had reached. My wife, Marci, and I took him to many specialists and had him undergo many therapies. Although no one would tell us directly what he suffered from, it became obvious that he had special needs.

When he failed to make any further progress despite the many interventions that were attempted, we were told to let Josh mature and learn as best he could at his own pace. Up to this point, Joshua could not read, write, or effectively communicate. His speech therapist was recommending the use of picture cards as a form of communication with others. I decided that the only option that I had was to teach him to be functional myself. This is what a good father does, and so the journey began.

I spent a long time working with him without making progress. Perhaps it was because I was trying to teach him to learn the traditional way that I was taught to learn. It was then that I embarked on teaching him to learn in a different way. This method was based on my clinical observation that many individuals with special needs have a significant impairment of their conscious thought process. This is the reason why these children have such a hard time learning using traditional education teaching methods. When these methods are used and are not found to be effective, the child is left behind until the child "matures" enough to learn once more. The word "matures" is a code-word that means we are unable to help your child any more. What so many experts fail to realize is that there is another way to learn when the conscious thought process is impaired.  These children can still be taught to learn by teaching and programming the subconscious thought process.

This is an innovative and novel way to learn. It makes sense that if our conscious thought process is impaired, then we should focus our efforts on the subconscious thought process that still has the ability to function normally. The only roadblock to doing so is that we have to first bypass conscious thought in order to have access to the subconscious mind.

Over time, I was able to independently develop a way that allowed me to succeed in bypassing conscious thought so that I could teach my son. The results were spectacular. He was able to finally learn. When we teach in this fashion, we can essentially program the subconscious mind to create a photographic memory.

Using what I had learned from my son, I began to understand that the dysfunctions that the patients in my medical practice exhibited were also related to a brain that refuses to allow itself to get better. The only difference is that all the patients who I saw and treated did not have an ongoing functional impairment of their conscious thought process that is present in those with special needs. The conscious thought process of these individuals was intact, yet their brains were refusing to allow them to heal and overcome the illness, physical trauma, or emotional injury that affected them. From the time and effort that I spent attempting to help my son, I recognized that the specific area of dysfunction was occurring in the subconscious thought process. This dysfunction is characterized by a brain that is continually and instinctually responding in a manner that does not benefit the individual. This form of brain injury is also directly responsible for many of the symptoms that people experience which fail to improve despite time and treatment. I have termed this type of brain dysfunction as nonstructural brain injury.

**This injury can be easily understood as a brain that is continuously responding in a nonbeneficial manner but is unable to consciously recognize or correct the defective instinctual response pattern.**

The research with my son had provided me with the foundation that I would use to attempt to correct the way the subconscious brain was abnormally responding in the patients I treat in my practice. My work with Josh taught me that the subconscious brain thinks and functions in concrete terms. This part of the brain can also be taught to respond so that a person can override a defective conscious thought process. The result is that it is possible to retrain the brain to respond in a beneficial manner.

I was first given an opportunity to see if this was so when an individual presented with a severe case of fibromyalgia. Her symptoms included constant soreness, squeezing pain sensations, pain to touch and pressure, as well as multiple trigger points. I treated her, and her symptoms went away and had not returned when I followed up with her several months later. I found similar success treating a number of other illnesses and injuries.

### The Principle Of Uniform Brain Response

At this point, I realized that the reason why multiple unrelated injuries and illnesses all successfully responded to a similar treatment is that the brain does not care what the actual injury or illness is that it is responding to. This is because the brain responds in a consistent and uniform fashion regardless of the injury that challenges it. It uses the same essential pathway. This makes sense from a developmental point of view because it would not be very feasible for the brain to use a trillion different pathways to deal with a trillion different challenges. In order for the brain to function efficiently, it needs to use one essential pathway that can be modified to handle the different challenges that represent a potential loss of control. This is a significant discovery because it implies that illness, physical trauma, and emotional injury are all related by this common pathway. This pathway and the principles relating how it applies to a broad spectrum of medical conditions are outlined in detail in the chapters of this book.

Over time, I continued to see and successfully treat more individuals. I began to realize that this form of brain injury is extremely common because it is seldom recognized or treated. When we consider that a nonstructural brain injury is present along with our other medical conditions, we are able to greatly expand our ability to diagnose and potentially treat many individuals.

There are no formal references for this book. It is based on my clinical experiences at work, my family experiences at home, and those from whom I have had the opportunity to learn in life. I would be remiss if I did not acknowledge the special individuals who helped make this possible. These include my wife, Marci, who is my partner and best friend. Two other individuals who are very important are my daughters Mindy and Amy, who have listened to my ideas and provided valuable contributions and feedback. The drive and inspiration for this book is my son, Joshua, who continues to teach those who will listen each and every day. I would also like to acknowledge my parents, Dorothy and Jack Herman, who allowed me to grow up in a loving house full of morals and ethical values.

Other very important individuals who have had an impact on the way I think and view this subject include Arnold and Anita Levin, Stuart, Gregg, and Adam Herman, Frank Garfield, Cheryl Beshada, Dennis Prager, Joseph Telushkin, Berel Wein, Dr. Harvey Roth, Dr. Lee Pravder, and Dr. Adam Cooper. I would like to personally thank Professor Barry Levine for the time and care he put into editing this manuscript.

# CHAPTER 1

*A New Understanding*

Jenny came to see me five months after she suffered a stroke. This injury left her with an extremely weak grip and difficulty ambulating. It appeared that the muscles in her foot were so weak that it caused her foot to drag on the floor when she attempted to walk. Her brain obviously suffered from an injury due to the stroke that left her unable to function as she used to. Since the usual medical treatments and rehabilitation failed to provide further improvement, she was left on her own to heal over time. I saw Jenny for an unrelated medical issue. After I heard of the symptoms that she was experiencing due to the stroke, I stated to her the seemingly impossible. I told her that her symptoms could be easily treated. My statement was based on the clinical understanding of how her brain functions and reacts. In Jenny's case, her brain was preventing her from improving.

## Introducing A Universal Medical Approach

As a physician, I continue to work to help the many Jennies of the world make significant clinical improvement that is not even considered possible by many other medical specialists. I am able to offer this treatment based on my understanding of the way the brain clinically reacts and responds. This field of clinical practice is termed **Neuroreactive Medicine**. Using this medical approach, a clinician can go beyond traditional medical diagnosis and effectively address the underlying reasons why a person's brain prevents him or her from clinically improving.

In order to appreciate how this approach can impact an individual's life, it is important to understand how the brain clinically functions. This new understanding will change the way we think about the symptoms that we experience.

To many of us, the brain is just a term that refers to the part of the body that is made up of a bunch of cells and nerves that extend and connect to the rest of the body. It is also viewed as the source of thought and decision making. A more functional description is found in the following statement.

**Our brains are composed of two important parts, a structural portion and a nonstructural portion.**

### The Structural Brain

The structural portion is the actual physical brain and surrounding nerves that we would see if we could look inside the skull or could visualize them on a CAT scan or MRI. If this portion is injured, then we would expect to see the effects of this injury in the way that we clinically function. We would anticipate that a more significant injury would result in greater physical dysfunction. An example is the patient described above. Jenny injured a portion of her brain and now suffers from foot drop and poor grip strength.

Since the brain is surrounded by a person's skull, a structural injury is challenging to treat because it is difficult to gain direct physical access to the brain itself. Frequently, all that is offered is rehabilitation, medication, and the hope that the patient's symptoms will improve over time. Unfortunately, this is not enough to address the needs of many individuals who suffer from such injuries. I have found that additional clinical improvement can be achieved when the diagnosis of a structural injury is reinterpreted using a neuroreactive medical approach. This innovative way of understanding brain dysfunction challenges the traditional way of thinking that a single structural injury, resulting from illness or trauma, is responsible for the symptoms that we experience. Based on my clinical experience in successfully treating individuals who suffer from stroke, neuropathy, and brain injury, I have come to a completely different and revolutionary discovery. This is stated as the following neuroreactive principle:

**There is not just one single structural injury responsible for many of the symptoms that a person suffers from. There are two injuries.**

**The first injury is the actual structural illness or physical trauma that was experienced.**

**The second injury is how the nonstructural brain was affected by the initial structural injury.**

The significance of this discovery is life changing. We can greatly improve the lives of many individuals who were previously under diagnosed and under treated. This leads us to the next neuroreactive principle.

**The percentage of symptoms due to structural injury and the percentage of symptoms due to nonstructural injury equals one hundred percent of symptoms that are experienced.**

While it may not be possible to treat the symptoms resulting from structural injury, it is completely possible to eliminate the symptoms resulting from the way the nonstructural brain was injured and incorrectly responded to the initial structural injury.

**The benefit of this approach is the ability to diagnose what percentage of an individual's symptoms is due to actual structural causes and what percentage is due to nonstructural causes.**

This is important because we can determine a person's potential to improve when we know exactly what percentage is due to nonstructural causes. For example, if twenty percent of a person's dysfunction resulting from a stroke is due to structural injury, then we can expect an eighty percent improvement in that person. If a nonstructural cause is responsible for ninety percent of a person's neuropathy, then we can expect that same individual to recover ninety percent after treatment. It is this ability to recognize and successfully treat nonstructural injury that allows my patients to get better when all hope has faded. To learn how this is possible, it is important to understand how the nonstructural brain functions.

### The Nonstructural Brain

The nonstructural brain is the portion that would not be seen if we were to look at an anatomic model or an imaging study. This is the part of the brain that thinks, remembers, and deals with making sure that our bodies function properly. You can think of it as the control or command center of the body. The subconscious mind is in charge of learning new information, making decisions, and responding to potential threats to the body's well being. It is also in charge of the ability to make changes as well as the storage and recall of memory. An examination the nonstructural brain reveals that it is composed of two main parts: the conscious mind and the subconscious mind. Both of these parts play a very critical role in contributing to a person's ongoing symptoms that were simply ignored or mistakenly attributed to a structural injury or illness.

I will now explain not only how the nonstructural brain functions to directly affect the way you feel, but also how this portion of the brain prevents you from getting better.

### How The Nonstructural Brain Functions

The nonstructural brain has the ability to adapt when faced with potential challenges to its well being. It may do so with ongoing normal function, or it may do so in a nonfunctional or impaired way, leading to clinical dysfunction.

This concept is illustrated by the way we allow the brain to change when we learn. If the brain were rigid, we would be robots, and we know that we are not robots. If our minds weren't able to adjust and learn new things, then one plus one would equal three. One plus one only equals the number two after our brains adapt to think and use the same vocabulary as everyone else around us.

Our nonstructural brains constantly change so that we can interact with others by learning as well as adapting to our environment. The nonstructural brain has an ongoing need to learn new responses in order to overcome stress and to stay in control. It also keeps us healthy by avoiding potential injury that may contribute to the symptoms we experience. As we grow older, we are constantly required to respond to new obstacles. In order to survive, our brains have to change both at the functional and cellular level. One can't be a functional adult if he or she cannot outgrow the mentality and the mindset of a child. The nonstructural brain has to change and adapt at each stage of our growth. It has to be able to meet our responsibilities as well as our environmental, social, and physical challenges. When we lose control due to an injury or illness, a portion of our nonstructural brain becomes unable to function as it should.

## An Analogy Showing How The Subconscious Mind Functions

The concept of how the conscious mind and the subconscious mind function can be understood using a computer analogy. Think of the brain as a type of super computer in which the subconscious memory is the hard drive. In order for the hard drive to work, it has to be connected and properly wired. These connections and intricate wirings have been previously described as the anatomical or structural brain. The subconscious memory, or hard drive, has to learn information, so it needs to be programmed. Once programmed, the information is stored until it needs to be recalled or used to execute a function to enable the computer to work properly. The hard drive, or subconscious memory, will function more efficiently and avoid potential losses of control when it learns new ways to respond. It also has the ability to change by erasing or overwriting old knowledge as well as by relearning through the use of software updates.

Just like ourselves, our computers also suffer and have to deal with stress, including constant potential external attacks on their well-being. Failure to effectively deal with these challenges will cause the computer to be affected in a negative way. The hard drive, just like our brain's subconscious memory, does not want to be permanently damaged. The result would be that it could not help the rest of the computer (our bodies) function correctly. To prevent this, the subconscious mind needs to be protected so that outside influences cannot permanently disrupt its vital functioning. To accomplish this, the hard drive employs a defense shield called a security program, or antiviral program, that is analogous to our conscious minds. The purpose of this software program called "the conscious mind" is to take over the subconscious memory or hard drive's day-to-day functions by making decisions and prohibiting access to the hard drive. Its role is to prevent outside undesirable forces from causing injury to the subconscious memory or hard drive.

This function of the conscious mind is similar to how we view the purpose of the pieces in a game of chess. In the game of chess, the role of all support pieces is to prevent the king from being affected by a constant external threat, the opponent's chess pieces. Our conscious mind functions in an identical manner in defense of our subconscious mind.

It is not that we are computers; it's that computers were designed to mimic the way our nonstructural brains are set up and clinically function. It is up to each of us to decide whether this design occurred as a coincidence or not.

### The Brain's Chain Of Command

There is also a chain of command that needs to be understood. When the nonstructural brain needs to make a decision or respond, it doesn't want to argue with itself. To prevent this from occurring, the subconscious memory is dominant over the conscious portion. The subconscious brain is also the source of infinite knowledge as well being as the ultimate decision making authority.

The conscious memory's role is to be the security guard for the subconscious memory. The purpose of the conscious mind is to use the knowledge, preferences, and judgments that it can understand from the subconscious memory in order to make functional decisions and run the body's day-to-day operations. If the conscious mind loses control, cannot make a decision, becomes confused, or has a question, it will defer the problem to the subconscious mind to make the final decision.

The subconscious mind is always present in the background waiting to intervene, if necessary. When things run smoothly, the subconscious mind is more resistant to suggestions. This is because if it isn't broken, then there is no perceived need to mentally fix it. When the subconscious mind experiences difficulty dealing with a situation, it is more amenable to change so that the body will not have to experience discomfort. It is able to adapt by being open to suggestions as well as by erasing defective memories. The subconscious mind also is receptive to learning new instinctual responses that will help improve the way it and the body functions. This process is similar to a computer getting a software update. The subconscious mind will also readily embrace new software or ideas that it perceives to be beneficial as long as they do not violate its morals or values.

## The Simplicity Of The Neuroreactive Approach

You do not need to know every anatomical and scientific detail concerning brain function in order to enable an individual to clinically improve.

## An example:

Imagine the new flat screen television on your wall. Do you know anything about how the TV works, how its parts are made, or how they function through intricate microcircuits to produce the picture that you can see? The answer is no. All you know is that your flat screen is high definition, the size in inches, and how much you paid for it. This last point is especially true since you got a great deal when you bought it. Are the internal details about how it works important? They are not. Why is this so? The details are unimportant because you know how to functionally make the TV do what you want to it do. You have the ability to maintain control and be in charge of how it responds. This is so because you know how to work the remote control.

This is similar to what can be done to help individuals get better by treating them using a neuroreactive medical approach. By employing this method of treatment, you can switch things on and you can switch things off. When one channel is acting out or showing things that are inappropriate, you can always switch to a more appropriate channel as well as block stations that are not suitable for normal functioning. You can even reprogram how the TV will respond to commands or signals. The neuroreactive principles in this book can be used to effectively treat individuals similar to the way that a remote control can correct an improperly functioning television. This treatment method allows the nonstructural brain to adapt in order to overcome many of the symptoms and dysfunctions you suffer from. These include the way your brain is preventing itself from getting better.

This area of clinical medicine does not deal with how things are anatomically located or wired. Neuroreactive medicine explains how the brain functions and instinctively responds to challenges that include the effect of illness, physical injury, and emotional dysfunction.

### The Injury That Prevents Our Brain From Getting Better

Neuroreactive medicine is especially beneficial in effectively treating nonstructural brain injury characterized by nonbeneficial instinctual responses. This type of injury occurs in the subconscious mind when it is unable to overcome a challenge that affects the body's ability to function the way it should.

You may mistakenly believe that this injury could not remotely apply to you. Once you discover how your illness or trauma contributed to the development of a medical condition known as a nonstructural brain injury, you will understand that your symptoms are directly related to this form of injury. These statements deeply challenge the way we are taught to think about the way our bodies function and respond to disease. This is especially true concerning those illnesses, injuries, and chronic dysfunctions that prevent us from structurally moving and feeling the way we should.

When we suffer from conditions such as pain, stroke, fibromyalgia, multiple sclerosis, neuropathy, neuralgias, amnesia, lameness, accidental injury, physical injury and trauma, fatigue, joint pain, and musculoskeletal dysfunction, we think of the diagnosis itself being responsible for the symptoms we experience. This is even more believable if the place on the body where the dysfunction occurs is an arm or a leg and is nowhere near the brain at all. What we mistakenly focus on is removing the pain and hurt at the place where our body is signaling us that something is wrong. We frequently fail to make the improvement that we need to feel better despite our best attempts. Many of us feel that we are only as good as the last pill that we took. Even when we take that pill, we often do not even come close to feeling as well as we remember feeling before we suffered our dysfunction.

It is time to rethink the way we view what ails us. When we remember that there is not just one single structural injury responsible for many of the symptoms that we suffer from, the neuroreactive approach starts to make a lot of sense. Using this innovative approach, we have an opportunity to determine whether a nonstructural injury may also be present and is preventing us from improving. This is done by learning how these long term nonstructural brain injuries and nonbeneficial instinctual responses develop and are formed in the subconscious mind.

# CHAPTER 2

*Neuroreactive Injury Formation*

### The Instinctual Response

We all make choices reflected by the way that we respond. Some of our choices benefit us and some fail to provide any meaningful good. This leads us to contemplate how much we are actually in control of who we are and how we function. We may even find ourselves reacting in ways that we would never have thought appropriate. After all, why would we knowingly do anything not in our best interest? The underlying reason for responding inappropriately may be due to a brain that refuses to allow itself to get better.

The answer to why we respond in the manner we do is deeply hidden in the way that our minds function. If we remove the decisions that are accomplished using our conscious awareness, we are left with the structured and predictable way that we unconsciously react. This functioning occurs every second of our existence in our subconscious brain whose purpose is to make sure that the body is working properly.

**The subconscious mind accomplishes this using instinctual reactions.**

These reactions constitute decisions that are initiated to promote one's well being and ongoing safety or to respond to a potential challenge that may lead to a loss of control. These instinctual reactions take precedence over and bypass the conscious thought process. The advantage of instinctually responding is that we can gain the ability to predictably respond and react quickly to a given stimulus or trigger.

This concept is easy to understand when you think of the last time you suddenly heard a buzzing sound right next to your ear. What did you do? Did you spend the time to ponder the complexities of what that sound may actually represent and how the vibrations of the buzzing produced a mild breeze wafting softly against your ear? You immediately reacted, didn't you? Your subconscious mind instinctively reacted by instantly triggering a pathway of events leading to an immediate response, which was shooing the source of the buzzing sound away before you were potentially stung. Other individuals have a slightly different instinctual response. They have the urge to instantly run as fast and as far as a track star running a 500-yard dash. The reason for this instinctual response is obvious. The individuals who are able to respond the fastest are ones who are the least likely to get injured or stung. The ability to respond this way is critical for those who may have a life threatening allergic reaction to a bee sting.

Another slightly humorous example is one which you may have actually experienced. It is very easy to replicate and leads to a protective instinctual response even when the person clearly understands that there is no real threat or imminent danger. All you have to do is walk up to a person sitting at his or her desk at work and casually discuss that you heard that there is a head lice outbreak. After you walk away and wait a couple of minutes, sneak up behind the person once more and gently move a few hairs on the back of his or her head. Now watch what happens. The person will instinctively overreact to your prior suggestion that there is a severe lice outbreak by scratching his or her head. It is humorous to watch, in a childish sort of way. You would think that once you perform this trick, the subject would be consciously aware and not instinctually respond, but often you can elicit the same instinctual response repeatedly throughout the day. This example is not discussed just so that you can find new ways to overcome boredom in the work environment. This simple experiment goes beyond annoying your coworkers by allowing you to examine how the subconscious brain predictably functions.

In each of these examples, there was a triggering event that led to an instant instinctual and predictable reaction. In fact, our brains are programmed with these and countless other instinctual reactions designed to benefit our well being.

**Two Distinct Instinctual Reactions**

This field of medicine takes this understanding of instinctual reactions and goes one step further. It recognizes that although our brains believe that our instinctual reactions are all designed to help us, this is not the case. This is shown in the following neuroreactive principle.

**There are two types of instinctual reactions, those that benefit us and those that do not.**

Examples of those that provide an advantage to us are the ones that allow us to maintain control and prevent us from suffering injury. These include the ability to effectively deal with stress and heal from illness.

The second category of instinctual reactions are the ones that do not benefit us. They are the reactions that are responsible for a brain that prevents itself from recovering. These negative instinctual reactions occur when we are unable to correctly respond to a potential challenge. Once present they will continue to contribute to the dysfunction you experience until they are addressed and removed.

Neuroreactive medicine is able to help you get better by recognizing that these negative instinctual responses are contributing to the clinical dysfunction or symptoms that you experience. Using this approach, you can experience significant clinical improvement when further progress is not considered medically possible. You can regain movement after a stroke. You can eliminate the symptoms of fibromyalgia, as well as a host of other conditions. Most importantly, you can gain the opportunity to get better. Using a neuroreactive approach, you will learn that many medical conditions which are traditionally thought of as purely physical or structural may not be entirely physical or structural at all. In fact, you will discover that these seemingly purely structural clinical conditions are actually composed of two separate components. The first component, a structural one, is located where it hurts or where the actual injury occurred. The second one is a nonstructural one which is located in the subconscious mind.

### Neuroreactive Challenges

There are three common types of potential neuroreactive challenges that the subconscious mind needs to overcome to prevent the formation of a nonbeneficial instinctual response. These challenges are the ones that may be present when we experience illness, physical trauma, and/or emotional dysfunction. The injuries that are experienced from these three common causes are often treated quite differently by clinicians if the diagnosis is perceived as a medical issue, a surgical issue, or even one of those "psychiatric issues."

It does not clinically matter which specific type of challenge the subconscious mind was unable to overcome that led to the formation of a nonbeneficial instinctual response. The subconscious mind responds the same and uses the same essential pathway to prevent a loss of control from occurring.

**The idea that the subconscious mind reacts in a single, unified pathway rather than in multiple different pathways is a very practical way to view how the brain functions.**

When the subconscious mind's function is approached in this fashion, the essential pathway remains the same because it can be adjusted to accommodate the underlying challenge regardless of its source.

I will now review the essential pathways that the brain follows to overcome a potential challenge leading to a loss of control. I will demonstrate how the subconscious mind develops a nonbeneficial instinctual response when it is unable to react in the appropriate manner. In this chapter, these pathways will be discussed in terms of medical illness or disease. In subsequent chapters, I will reveal how the same essential pathways can also apply to physical trauma and emotional dysfunction.

It is important to understand how the subconscious mind is able to overcome the effect of disease or illness without developing an inappropriate instinctual response. This is seen in the following pathway.

**The Neuroreactive Pathway Demonstrating The Successful Ability Of The Subconscious Mind To React And Respond**

Illness or disease process affecting the body

↓

Produces symptoms and dysfunction at the site of the injury or occurrence

↓

This signals and challenges the nonstructural brain to respond to the symptoms and dysfunction so that a temporary state of loss of control occurs in the subconscious mind. This is termed

↓

Nonstructural brain confusion

This term reflects the brain's ability to respond to and overcome the loss of control due to the symptoms or dysfunction caused by the disease or illness.

↓

The illness resolves with or without treatment or the brain is able to regain control.

↓

This leads to recovery and continued normal functioning of the nonstructural brain.

The above pathway demonstrates the basic steps that occur each day in our lives. We are frequently unaware of what is going on since many of our instinctual responses are determined by our present understanding of the potential challenge we face and our past experiences. When we are able to correctly respond and prevent the development of a nonbeneficial instinctual response, our subconscious minds simply stay in control so that we do not experience any ongoing symptoms and dysfunction resulting from the disease.

When dealing with an illness or a disease process that is present in the body, it is critical to remember that the illness or disease is not limited to only producing symptoms at the site where it hurts. The disease or illness can negatively affect the nonstructural brain as well. Now, let's look at a pathway that shows what can occur when the brain is unable to overcome or properly respond to injury, dysfunction, or symptoms resulting from a disease or illness.

**The Neuroreactive Pathway Demonstrating The Formation Of A Nonbeneficial Response When The Subconscious Mind Is Unable To React And Respond**

Illness or disease process affecting the body

Produces symptoms and dysfunction at the site of the injury or occurrence

That signals and challenges the nonstructural brain to respond to the symptoms and dysfunction so that a temporary state of loss of control occurs in the subconscious mind. This is termed

↓

Nonstructural brain confusion

This reflects the brain's ability to respond to and overcome the loss of control due to the symptoms or dysfunction caused by the disease or illness.

Despite treatment, the subconscious, nonstructural brain is unable to completely resolve the loss of control.

↓

Instinctual imprinting occurs

This results in some portions of the subconscious, nonstructural brain staying in control and remaining unaltered and unaffected by the disease.

Other portions of the subconscious, nonstructural brain are now over-ridden or reprogrammed by the process of instinctual imprinting. This leads to the formation of a…

↓

Nonstructural brain injury

A nonstructural brain injury occurs due to the inability of the subconscious, nonstructural brain to resolve the loss of control and the subsequent negative instinctual imprinting that occurs.

↓

The result of this type of injury is that a nonbeneficial instinctual response is formed. From this point on, the portion of the subconscious mind that was injured will respond in an inappropriate way.

↓

This type of injury may be clinically recognizable by abnormal or undesirable side effects, symptoms, or behavioral changes. These nonbeneficial changes can significantly contribute as a percentage to a person's overall illness or disease.

↓

Once a nonstructural brain injury or nonbeneficial instinctual response is recognized, it can usually be treated successfully. Thus, the percentage that the nonbeneficial instinctual response contributed to a person's overall illness or disease can be eliminated. Many times this results in significant and noticeable clinical improvement.

The pathways in the above paragraphs are extremely important in expanding our understanding of how disease or illness can negatively affect the nonstructural brain. This pathway differs from the earlier pathway because the nonstructural brain is unable to completely resolve the loss of control despite treatment.

These pathways show that we instinctively react in a predictable manner based on the way our subconscious mind responded to a current or past challenge. These reactions result in the clinical symptoms you experience. Each day, I am able to clinically identify individuals who continue to suffer from such injuries. These are individuals whose brains refuse to allow them to get better. There is no shortage of these individuals, since the majority of these people have never been correctly diagnosed or treated. It always amazes me how many individuals there are that can clearly benefit from appropriate treatment directed at the source of their dysfunction.

# CHAPTER 3

*Exploring Treatments That Can Help You Get Better*

When people experience illness or suffer pain, they frequently turn to their doctor for answers. The patient tells the physician what he or she perceives as being wrong as well as the pertinent history associated with the problem. After a history is taken and all the test results are in, a diagnosis may be rendered and a treatment pathway recommended. There are four commonly used treatment pathways. These are: expectant, surgical, medical, and "I don't know." When dealing with the diagnosis of nonbeneficial instinctual responses, it is important to evaluate these therapeutic options from a neuroreactive perspective to see if these treatments can provide the ability to improve.

**Expectant treatment**

Expectant treatment refers to following the patient's condition without any type of medical or surgical intervention. Such medical conditions will usually resolve by themselves or will remain without negatively affecting a person. These conditions include symptoms for which further therapy is needed but not available. These individuals have tried all the usual treatments, including the newest and most popular ones. Unfortunately, they do not improve or get better. They are frequently left with the choice of living with what they suffer from or seeking a different approach to the diagnosis and treatment of what ails them. They eventually get tired of just putting up with their dysfunction, so they are continually on the lookout for something that can help them get better. The opportunity to help these people exists when we consider that many of their symptoms may be due to nonstructural injury. Some common examples of conditions that have a nonstructural component include stroke, chronic pain, phantom pain, post traumatic stress, neuropathy, and especially fibromyalgia. These people do not improve because the treatments that they have tried did not target the way the nonstructural brain responded to their illness or injury.

### Surgical Treatment

Surgical intervention involves treatment through the performance of a procedure or operation. If there is a structural problem, mass, or something deemed to be broken, then surgery is a way of fixing it. From a neuroreactive perspective, surgery can remedy a structural issue, but it cannot treat the way the brain was unable to respond to a potential loss of control precipitated by the illness or trauma. Any symptoms due to nonstructural issues that are present will persist despite successful surgical intervention. A few examples include nonspecific persistent pain, hypersensitivity, numbness, and neuropathy.

Serious consideration should be given that a nonstructural injury is present when one experiences ongoing pain or loses the ability to fully move an extremity, especially after a surgery that was deemed successful. An example of this is experiencing the symptoms of pain and loss of range of motion after undergoing successful rotator cuff surgery. Many individuals can be effectively treated when these issues are addressed using a neuroreactive medical approach.

### Medical Treatment

This involves overcoming a condition through the use of behavioral modification, such as diet, exercise, weight loss, or stopping smoking. Medical therapy also involves the use of medication in order to treat an illness or disease. The abundant availability of pills for every condition can lead to the tendency of many physicians to overly rely on pills to overcome a patient's illness and suffering. The goal of prescribing is based on finding a pill that can work to remove the symptoms of disease. The benefits of the medication must outweigh the side effects associated with it. Certain medications are curative. An example is an antibiotic that is used to treat a bladder infection that will eliminate the causative bacteria. Unfortunately, many medications are not curative but are a type of Band-Aid that serves to control the symptoms of a disease. Examples include blood pressure pills to temporarily reduce blood pressure or pain pills which are used to control chronic pain. These medications are only as good as the last pill taken. Once the beneficial effect of the pill wears off, the patient will be back to where he started.

### Treatments Titled "I Don't Know"

This form of communication occurs if the medication, surgery, or medical management cannot help a person overcome the symptoms of chronic disease. When this occurs, the patient is informed that no effective treatment has yet been developed, or simply, "I don't know." Many times this is conveyed through the following words, "Keep taking the medication (usually at a higher dosage) and let's see what happens, there is nothing more that can be done, or let's give it more time." When this occurs, the patient is left on his or her own to live with the condition as well as its daily symptoms, which frequently include pain and limited mobility. These symptoms are frequently disabling and hinder many people from achieving their full potential in life. Even worse, there are additional obstacles that need to be overcome, including the possibility being classified as a person who cannot be treated.

### The Psychosomatic or Psychogenic Myth

When many people who expect to get better fail to do so, they are told that their symptoms are psychosomatic, psychogenic, or that "you just made up the symptoms in your mind." Some people are even told that they are "crazy." The health care practitioners who say these words are doing a great disservice. Several clinicians use the word psychosomatic or psychogenic to send a secret message to their patients. This hidden message can be decoded in everyday layman's terms to mean, "I cannot help you." It's true. If a clinician tells someone that he or she cannot be helped, it is up to the sufferer to begin to look elsewhere. It's not that these clinicians do not want to help; it's just that they are not familiar with an area of medicine that may help you overcome what you are suffering from. These practitioners just do not know how to treat your symptoms, nor do they know where to refer you.

When a healthcare practitioner says that the symptoms are psycho-somatic or psychogenic, he or she is implying an even bigger disservice and diagnostic error. This person is blaming the patient for consciously causing his or her own symptoms. The clinician is implying that the patient can overcome the symptoms if he or she really wanted to and that this individual knows why the symptoms are present. These same practitioners may suggest that the patient is deriving some benefit from the suffering. Some bolder medical caregivers may even make accusations of malingering. If you are not deriving a benefit from your suffering, you may feel very disheartened when someone makes this accusation. The fact is that you can't consciously help yourself. Which would you rather do, continue to suffer and experience pain or have the ability to overcome your illness and get much better? To me and many others, it's a no-brainer.

When given the choice, most people want to overcome their dysfunction and feel good again. Most people would do it in a second. The journey through life is hard enough without having to suffer additionally due to one's medical and personal issues.

We may ask ourselves why many individuals who are labeled psychosomatic cannot help themselves. The answer is that many individuals are unable to help themselves because the problem, or nonbeneficial instinctual response that causes their symptoms, cannot be found by the conscious mind. To aid in our understanding of why it is difficult for the conscious mind to determine the source of the dysfunctional response located in the subconscious mind, let us reexamine how the conscious thought process neuroreactively functions.

**How the Conscious Thought Process Functions**

We initially learned that the conscious mind is the part of the nonstructural brain that one uses to think, function, make decisions, and react to the stresses of everyday events. It also blindly follows the decisions made by the controlling and authoritative subconscious mind; the conscious mind usually does not question the subconscious mind or seek to understand exactly how or why a decision was made. It only understands that once a decision is made in the subconscious mind, the conscious mind will respond in a very predictable fashion to carry out that decision.  This is because the conscious mind knows that the subconscious mind's job is to never knowingly make a decision that would result in any type of hurt, injury, or dysfunction to a person's well being. The conscious mind blindly follows the decisions established by the subconscious mind that result in many individuals being unable help themselves even if they wanted to. This is especially true when a person experiences symptoms or dysfunction due to an instinctual response that does not particularly benefit him or her.

**When such an abnormal instinctual response occurs, these individuals are continually symptomatic because their conscious minds fail to question whether or not the instinctual response made by the subconscious mind is truly beneficial.**

These individuals are completely unaware that they are reacting to a previous event that occurred when the subconscious mind was challenged and was overwhelmed, leading to a loss of control. Often, these nonbeneficial instinctual reactions may have been present for many years.  This creates the clinical situation where one has matured and gone on with his or her life, but the subconscious mind is stuck reacting to the past. Thus, it is very understandable that an affected symptomatic person would find it very difficult to consciously overcome what he or she is unaware of. Most can only work to successfully overcome issues that they know are present. They only know that they continue to suffer or react in a negative way to an event without the conscious ability to know why this is occurring. This understanding can provide many people the answer they seek as to why they are unable to help themselves.

**Other Medical Treatments**

Other treatments used to overcome issues of the conscious and subconscious mind are based on a different understanding of how dysfunction of the subconscious mind affects a person's inner conflicts and the development of chronic life problems. These are known as psychotherapy and psychoanalysis. These therapies have benefited many individuals. The discussion of the exact way these therapies work, along with the vocabulary needed to clarify exactly what is being done, varies depending on the interpretive source.

The disadvantage of such an approach is that there has to be an extensive commitment on the part of the individual undergoing treatment. There is a need for multiple visits to achieve success, and it is not uncommon to require three to five sessions per week for two to five years. There is also the potential for considerable expense in which the cost per session varies depending on geographic region, expertise of the practitioner, and the time spent during each session. The monthly cost and the time away from work needed to attend these sessions may be prohibitive to many. There may be additional resistance by insurance and managed care plans to cover an ongoing expense that may last for a considerable period of time. It is important to note that the scope of these treatments is generally limited to psychiatric dysfunction. These therapies are not commonly used to treat perceived structural dysfunction that may include injury resulting from medical illness or physical trauma. For example, one would not expect that psychotherapy and psychoanalysis would allow a patient to regain movement of his arm after a stroke or remove the pain and pins and needles sensations in one's leg due to multiple sclerosis.

Up to this point, we have discussed treatments which maintain the status quo or are considered traditional. If these were sufficient, then everyone would be able to improve clinically, but this is not the case. What is needed is a more encompassing approach that is able to effectively treat nonstructural injury caused by illness, physical trauma, and emotional dysfunction. All of these categories of injury may be effectively addressed and successfully overcome through the neuroreactive medical principles outlined in this book.

### Directing Treatment at A Brain That Refuses To Get Better

In order to effectively treat the injuries that affect our subconscious minds, we need to identify what it is we are actually treating: **a brain that refuses to allow itself to get better.** This is the result of nonstructural brain injuries seen as instinctual responses that do not provide benefit and directly contribute to the symptoms we experience.

**The cornerstone of treatment is to realize the possibility that a nonstructural injury may be present and is affecting the individual in a nonbeneficial manner. In order to treat something, we first have to conclude that there is something to treat.**

### A Healthy Example

The following example will allow you to rethink your ability to identify which dysfunctions you experience are due to an actual physical or structural injury and which are due to nonbeneficial instinctual responses. This example will also benefit your health and demonstrate how we instinctively react without even realizing what we are doing.

A common goal of exercise is to achieve a certain level of fitness. For some people it involves a very high level of activity, and for others the level of intensity is not as pronounced. This is still good since some exercise is better than no exercise.

Many people perform a certain exercise for a set number of repetitions. An example of this is to do fifty sit ups in a row, or if one is really fit, one hundred. Individuals who can do this may notice that it is much easier to do the first ten than the last ten. Many will notice that it takes much more muscular effort and determination to accomplish those final few, especially if they challenge the individual's physical ability. Some people even dread getting to sit up number 35 because after that it is all an uphill crunch. Things get even more difficult after number 42; many find that they are using other muscle groups to compensate for those final ones.

We just assume that the final sit ups are telling us that it is an endurance and strength issue and that we need to be consistent and progressive in our workouts so we will achieve the ability to perform them effortlessly. What we really are assuming is that the difficulty encountered in performing the last 20 is a structural issue. This makes sense to us because that is why we are working out in the first place, to overcome the structural issues due to inactivity or underutilization of our potential. Since it is a structural issue, we need to overcome it with more exercise to increase our endurance and strength. After all, it would be difficult to improve without physical activity or effort.

There is an easier way. The next time you attempt to perform a set of fifty, I would like you to use a slightly different strategy and notice a remarkable difference.

Do a sit up and count out loud to yourself with each subsequent one.

Start at the beginning: 1, 2, 3…

When you get to the number 27, start counting backwards and continue to do the sit ups: 26, 25, 24…

When you get to the number 16, start counting upward from the number 12: for example, 12, 13, 14…

When you get to the number 18, start counting backwards by threes: 15, 12, 9, 6, 3, 1.

And you are done. You just did 50 sit ups.

When you exercise using this or a similar method of counting, you will be surprised at what you discover. You will find that you are able to do those fifty sit ups without the same discomfort or physical exertion that was needed when you did them by counting straight up from one to fifty. This exercise demonstrates that it was not a physical or structural issue that you needed to overcome. If it was, then you would still have had the same discomfort and physical exertion that would have been experienced by counting from one to fifty.

### How Can This Be Explained?

The answer is that the difficulty performing sit ups is due to the way the subconscious mind instinctually responds to the task of doing them. The task of doing sit ups is actually a series of instinctual reactions or responses emanating from the subconscious mind. It is based on the subconscious mind's imprinted learned response resulting from its perceived experience that took place when you first attempted your first few sets of fifty sit ups. The subconscious mind learned that sit ups numbers 1-26 were associated with feeling comfortable and exerting minimal effort, while the sit ups numbers 35-50 were associated with a negative perception which included exertion, difficulty, and effort. Your subconscious mind has been unconsciously programmed to instinctually respond to a trigger which are the numbers associated with an exercise.

### Developing Instinctual Responses

You are born with an initial set of beneficial instinctual responses and are unconsciously programmed along the way with additional ones that will contribute to your well being as you mature by learning and adapting. These responses allow your subconscious mind to maintain control so that you function the way that you should. What happens is that you are continually subjected to challenges that represent a potential loss of control of the ability of your subconscious mind to instinctually respond in a way that benefits you. In the previously outlined pathways, we recognized that disease and illness are two of the many common challenges that can potentially cause the subconscious mind to lose control. When your subconscious mind is unable to overcome these challenges, it is reprogrammed to instinctively respond in ways that do not benefit you. The result is that your subconscious mind becomes the sum of your beneficial and nonbeneficial instinctual responses. These nonbeneficial instinctual responses may contribute to the symptoms, illness, or behavioral changes that you clinically experience.

This is understood by the following neuroreactive principle.

**The clinical symptoms that you suffer from equal the sum of your**

**structural findings or physical disease**
**+**
**your conscious reactions**
**+**
**your beneficial subconscious instinctual reactions**
**+**
**your nonbeneficial subconscious instinctual reactions.**

Each of these parts contributes a certain percentage to the total disease process and the clinical symptoms you experience. Traditional medical thought has focused its effort on addressing just the structural findings, rather than acknowledging that there are other treatable factors that need to be considered.

### An Example Relating How We Are The Sum Of Our Structural And Nonstructural Parts

A parallel scenario may help you relate to this concept. Let's say your car is functioning inadequately. Your mechanic indicates that a part is not working correctly, so he replaces the part at considerable time and expense. After a few days, you discover that the car is slightly improved but does not function one hundred percent the way that it should. You then take more time off from work and bring the car back to be reevaluated. This time you are told that along with the seemingly defective part that was appropriately replaced there is an additional dysfunction. There seems to be a problem with the way the central computer in your car is functioning. It appears that the chip responsible for making sure that the structural part is firing properly is sending out the wrong signals. The mechanic relates to you that the dysfunction in your car appears to be a combination of a faulty program sending inappropriate responses in addition to the structural part that he previously replaced. If the computer in your car is not functioning correctly and is sending out improper responses, then it is unlikely that the car would clinically function the way that it optimally should. Fortunately, he tells you that all that is needed is a software update and your car will be function properly. Unfortunately, it still costs you an additional undisclosed amount of money for the diagnostic analysis and the software remedy. In other words, the way your car functions is the sum of its structural parts and the beneficial and nonbeneficial signals it receives to make the parts function properly. Obviously, humans are not cars. If we were, then everyone would want to be the high-end, red sports car, but the basic concept of how cars run properly mimics the way we function to a certain extent.

We need to take into account and clinically address the way that we instinctually respond because there may be significant under treatment when nonstructural injury is not addressed. Since the contributing percentages of these components make up the symptoms you experience from your illness or injury, it is not difficult to determine where improvement can be made. Most improvement can be made in the area of instinctual responses that do not benefit us. A goal of neuroreactive medical treatment is to reverse the clinical dysfunction caused by these nonbeneficial instinctual responses. This can be accomplished by eliminating the need for a nonbeneficial response to instinctually occur. Using the previous examples that were provided, it is similar to providing a software update when our hard drive or subconscious memory is not functioning the way that it should.

## Additional Neuroreactive Principles

It is useful to consider the following neuroreactive principles when dealing with the functioning of the subconscious mind.

1. The more individual nonbeneficial instinctual responses that are present, the more clinical dysfunction may be seen.

2. Some nonbeneficial instinctual responses may be more clinically apparent than others.

3. The sum of the nonbeneficial instinctual responses may be greater than the individual parts.

4. Multiple related individual nonbeneficial instinctual responses may produce more dysfunction than multiple unrelated individual nonbeneficial instinctual responses.

5. A greater of loss of control may lead to the formation of a greater nonbeneficial instinctual response, resulting in greater clinical dysfunction.

6. Not all areas of the subconscious mind are of equal noticeable clinical function. The greater that a potential loss of control affects a critical area of the subconscious mind's clinical functioning, the more likely a noticeable clinical nonbeneficial instinctual response will be present.

7. A single nonbeneficial instinctual response may result in either a single clinical response or multiple clinical responses that do not provide benefit.

8. The nonbeneficial instinctual response that may have appeared to "help" you overcome a potential loss of control in the past may negatively affect the ability to respond appropriately to subsequent future challenges.

All of these principles allow you to gain insight into the functioning of the subconscious mind, but if there is one overriding clinical pearl that can impact your life, it would be the following:

If it is possible to develop a nonbeneficial instinctual response, then it must be possible to remove the nonbeneficial instinctual response as well.

\* \* \*

**Communicating with the part of the brain that refuses to allow you to get better**

There are many ways to directly communicate with the subconscious brain.  Some are easily achieved and some require more effort to accomplish.  When we perceive that this task will be difficult, we are more likely to use an in-depth, overly complicated method with vague concepts and confusing vocabulary.  That is why the answer is never stumbled upon. Many well intentioned individuals try to make things appear complex when they do not have to be.  Complexity prevents us from obtaining a simple understanding and disguises the underlying truth.

The following neuroreactive principle allows this process to become a lot simpler and make much more sense.

**The subconscious mind will respond instinctually when it is presented with the correct trigger**.

If the desired instinctual response is to bypass the conscious thought process so that a clinician can communicate directly with the subconscious mind, all that needs to occur is for us to discover the appropriate trigger.

**In clinical practice, the simple words and behaviors which we use each day are the triggers that allow us to bypass the conscious memory's defenses so we can interact directly with the subconscious mind.**

Once we are able to bypass the conscious memory's defenses, we are able to use a neuroreactive approach to communicate directly with the subconscious memory in order to help that portion of the brain identify and overcome whatever nonstructural difficulty or potential loss of control the body is reacting to. Effective communication with the subconscious mind can enable it to overcome the nonstructural effects of negative imprinting from illness, physical trauma, and emotional dysfunction. When this is accomplished, the subconscious mind can once again function in a perfectly normal fashion.

Similar attempts to bypass conscious thought have been used in many fields, including psychiatry, psychology, hypnotherapy, neurolinguistic programming (NLP), as well as in meditation, prayer, relaxation, movies, music, and commercial televised advertising. Just remember the last time you had the impulsive urge to call in and purchase an unneeded item that looked appealing on TV.

**In clinical practice, the specific method that a practitioner uses to bypass conscious thought does not matter**.

This important principle is illustrated in the following example:

There was a race between three individuals to get to a finish line two miles away. The first person decided to walk. The second rode his bike and the third drove his sports car. If the goal was to reach the finish line which person would reach the finish line last?

In this example, the finish line represents the relaxation necessary to bypass the conscious thought process and the three individuals represent the available different methods used to trigger that relaxation. It is expected that all three individuals will reach the finish line so it does not matter which method is used. The only difference is how fast an individual's method will get him to the finish line.

A discussion of the merits concerning specific methods used by various clinicians is purposely omitted in this book. **The reason is that the method that is used is not important.** A comparative debate on the subject would only divert attention from the message of this book, the purpose of which is to show how your brain is preventing you from recovering.

This point is demonstrated in the following statement. You cannot open a locked door that will accept any key when you are stuck arguing which key is better than the others. It does not matter which key unlocks the door as long as you can gain access to what lies behind it.

Bypassing conscious thought is only the very beginning and can be thought of as similar to taking a taxi to your caregiver's office in order to get treated. The fact that you are now in a location where it is possible to be treated does not mean that you are treated. What matters clinically is what you are able to accomplish once you bypass conscious thought, because that is where the real treatment takes place.

Once a practitioner is successfully able to bypass the conscious thought process, neuroreactive treatment can be initiated. A successful approach to treating individuals is based on the understanding and the application of the neuroreactive principles outlined in this book. Treatment is accomplished by identifying and eliminating the nonstructural injury that produced an individual's nonbeneficial instinctual responses.

## A Typical Office Visit

Countless individuals go to see their health care practitioner without realizing that their chronic symptoms are due to nonstructural causes or a brain that prevents itself from recovering. Most of the time, these individuals are being seen for a completely unrelated reason, such as a yearly physical examination. I use the following approach to evaluate and treat the many patients I see with these types of maladies.

1. I listen to the patient's history and the issues that are brought up, as well as perform an exam that includes addressing the reason why the patient is seeing me.

2. I ask appropriate and related questions, including, "Which specialists have you seen and how have you been treated?" I also ask, "Are you any better as a result of the ongoing treatments and medications that you are taking?" The answer is almost universally "NO!" The typical clinical picture is a person who has experienced an illness, physical trauma, or emotional dysfunction a long time earlier. This individual still suffers from pain or other dysfunction without getting better despite years of treatment by many specialists, medications, rehabilitation, and time. This may sound very familiar to many who suffer or know of someone who suffers chronically.

3. I determine from the above history if it is possible that the patient's symptoms or dysfunction may be due to a nonstructural brain injury or nonbeneficial instinctual response.

4. If I am reasonably certain that a patient's symptoms or dysfunction may be due to such an injury, I will inform the patient that I feel that I can help him or her get better. The conversation usually goes something like this.

Doctor: By the way, did you know I can help you get rid of your symptoms?

Individuals who hear these words usually sit quietly for a moment, just staring at me. People frequently take a moment to digest the words they thought that they would never hear or even consider possible. The first thing that people usually do is look at my face to see if I am serious about what I just said to them. When they see that I am serious and that the tone of my voice reaffirms that I can help them, they will ask me the following question out of sheer disbelief. "How is it possible that you can treat these symptoms that do not get better despite years of treatment?" I explain that that even though the area where the dysfunction occurred has probably been treated and has recovered, the area in the nonstructural brain responsible for dealing with this injury has not recovered. The nonstructural brain has not been able to overcome the loss of control it experienced due the nonbeneficial way the brain reacted. As a result, the nonstructural brain is continually responding to the past injury in an abnormal fashion, even though the reason it needed to respond this way has probably long since disappeared. When this occurs, the brain is essentially refusing to allow an individual to get better. I then inform the patient that the correct diagnosis that would explain the symptoms would be a nonstructural injury.

I explain that this type of injury occurs in the part of the brain known as the subconscious mind. The subconscious mind is responsible for making sure the body functions the way it should even when an individual experiences illness, physical trauma, or emotional dysfunction. I then find it useful to briefly review "the computer analogy" with my patient. This comparison is easy to understand because it is simple and people can relate to it. The analogy goes as follows:

Just think of the hard drive in your computer as your subconscious mind. You know that when you take it out of the box for the first time, it runs perfectly. When you negatively affect your hard drive by letting your kids surf the Internet or download questionable files, you may notice that it does not function the way that it should. So I ask my patient, "How do you fix a hard drive that is abnormally reacting to something that it should not?" The patient usually does not respond and waits for me to speak. The answer is a software update. You fix a malfunctioning hard drive by giving it a software update or by retraining the brain to respond in a beneficial manner.

I explain that I can treat the issue in the subconscious mind that produced the nonbeneficial instinctual response. The whole process usually takes only a single visit for the patient to get better. In subsequent chapters you will see that it is possible to overcome a wide range of clinical symptoms and dysfunction that is not possible using only traditional medical treatment.

## Questions And Answers

I have found it clinically useful to use the following conversational responses to clarify what a neuroreactive medical approach is. In this way, I am able to not only meet but exceed the expectation of an individual who is considering treatment. Many of these responses are the answers to several of my patients' questions that have been raised over the years.

**Should I undergo neuroreactive treatment instead of traditional medical treatment?**

A neuroreactive approach only addresses the clinical symptoms and dysfunction due to nonbeneficial instinctual responses or nonstructural brain injury. It should be used in addition to appropriate conventional medical therapy. Many individuals seek a neuroreactive approach when they fail to respond to traditional medical treatment. The motivation for this is obvious. Why suffer clinically when you do not have to? If there is a method that can overcome a part of your injury or illness that is not addressed by a traditional medical approach, it just makes sense to get that treatment. This is especially true if your injury or illness is due to a nonstructural cause.

When a neuroreactive medical approach is applied, many untreatable clinical symptoms can be completely eliminated. This simple and effective method of treatment is based on the way the brain is programmed to instinctually react and respond. Neuroreactive therapy can also enhance a medical or surgical approach and lead to a faster recovery than simply providing the treatment alone.

**Will my clinical symptoms return once they are treated?**

The result of neuroreactive therapy is your clinical symptoms and dysfunction due to nonstructural brain injury should go away and stay away. The fact that your symptoms cease to exist after treatment supports the diagnosis that a nonstructural injury and not a physical or structural cause is responsible for those symptoms. Most people are expected to get better and stay better. These symptoms are not expected to return unless the subconscious mind is reinjured at a later date or if there is significant progression of a chronic illness in the future. This topic is discussed in detail in the chapter dealing with diabetic neuropathy.

**Can a neuroreactive medical approach provide a diagnosis of the percentage of my clinical symptoms due to actual illness or physical injury as opposed to the percentage due to nonstructural injury?**

This method of treatment is an efficient way to access the percentage of an individual's clinical symptoms due to actual structural disease and the percentage due to nonstructural causes. The symptoms that remain after treatment are due to actual structural injury. The most surprising finding is that neuroreactive medicine continually redefines what is structural as opposed to what is nonstructural illness and injury. Many of the clinical symptoms and dysfunctions that were attributed solely to structural causes can now be reinterpreted as being made up of a much larger percentage of treatable, nonstructural causes. This knowledge is critical to your well being because treatment can potentially reverse the percentage of your illness or disease that is due to these nonbeneficial instinctual responses.

**What do you say to individuals during treatment that allows them to get better?**

The most effective words are the simple truth. These words can enable a person's subconscious thought process to instinctively respond in a beneficial manner. The exact words needed to overcome a particular difficulty are individual and personalized to reflect the desired instinctual response. A published listing of these words and phrases would greatly diminish the caregiver's ability to bypass the critical conscious thought process. This would prevent a potential treatment from reaching the subconscious mind due to a heightened awareness and increased resistance of the conscious thought process. A treatment that is prevented from reaching its destination will be ineffective.

When you view a list of new valuable information, you are reading it with your conscious mind. Thus, you will reason and respond to this information through the process of conscious decision making. Your conscious mind will resist your ability to beneficially change by preventing the information from reaching the subconscious mind.

This is true because if you had the conscious ability to change, you would have done so a long time ago.

**A common example:**

Maintaining proper body weight is important for one's health. Imagine that you desired to communicate the beneficial goal to lose weight with the subconscious thought process but could not get past the critical conscious mind.

Caregiver: You should lose some weight.

Conscious thought process: Look who's talking. Why don't you lose a few pounds then maybe you could tell someone else to lose some weight. You weigh more than I. Let me see you pass up the pizza and chips for a few weeks, then tell me what to do.

It is the conscious mind's ability to recognize and critically respond that prevents the desired outcome of losing weight. This example reaffirms that it is difficult to subconsciously change when one can't get past the conscious thought process.

**Does neuroreactive treatment require any painful tests or needles?**

This method of treatment is completely painless and does not involve any tests, procedures, lab work, machines, or needles. All that is needed to retrain the brain to remove a nonbeneficial instinctual response is an effective communication approach.

**Will neuroreactive treatment interfere with any other treatment I may be undergoing?**

This common concern is frequently voiced. Neuroreactive medical treatment will not interfere or worsen any other treatment that you are undergoing. You can only benefit. This form of treatment simply provides an opportunity for an individual to overcome clinical dysfunction due to nonstructural injury. This approach is based on the way the brain functions. This method does not remove, disturb, or affect any instinctual responses that are beneficial to you. You can think of this treatment as removing the bad while leaving the good.

**Are there people who would not benefit from this method of treatment?**

Most individuals who seek treatment genuinely want to get better and feel better because they are tired of suffering or experiencing dysfunction. They are the ones who usually are successful and clinically improve. In clinical practice, I attempt to treat only honest and sincere people who I believe suffer from nonstructural injury. Those who do not meet this description will not improve and are encouraged to seek treatment elsewhere.

I have also identified a few individuals who will not likely benefit by undergoing treatment. These are people who I am unable to effectively communicate with due to a language barrier, those with a mental or cognitive impairment that prevents them from understanding or participating in treatment, and those who are unable to hear despite adjusting their hearing aids to the maximal volume possible. Others include those who only suffer from a structural issue and do not have any nonstructural injury. A person must want to participate and undergo treatment. I cannot treat someone against his or her wishes even if a loved one or guardian urges me to do so.

There are also some individuals that are okay with their symptoms or dysfunction even though everyone else around them is not. They do not perceive the need to overcome their illness because they do not believe that anything is wrong. These people deeply believe that if it is not broken, then there is no need to fix it. Once these individuals come to the understanding that something is broken, they can then be easily treated.

There is also a subset of individuals in any clinical population who, for one reason or another, do not want to get better. These are people who still derive a benefit from their addiction or rely on others to compensate for their clinical symptoms or significant psychiatric dysfunction. Some dishonest people resist being treated in order to collect damages in a lawsuit. Deep down inside, these individuals do not really want to improve at the present time. They do not want to take responsibility for their actions, their behaviors, their interactions with others, and their lives. They want to avoid dealing with their ongoing emotions and failures.

Other individuals who do not benefit from therapy are those who display ongoing conscious anger over a past issue that they do not want to overcome or resolve. These people choose to be manipulative and vindictive. They seek retribution through self destructive behavior and hurting those they believe to be responsible for way they feel. They are unable to forgive themselves or those who love them despite being asked for forgiveness. Even when a neuroreactive injury may be present and contribute to a person's overall dysfunction, there is a time and a place for everything. These individuals would benefit from counseling and a long term relationship with both a psychologist and psychiatrist. I have found that nonstructural injuries are more amenable to treatment once the anger issues have been professionally addressed.

**How many treatments are needed before I will be able to see clinical improvement?**

Usually only one treatment is needed to experience significant clinical improvement. This is especially true if the dysfunction or clinical symptoms are due to a single, nonbeneficial instinctual response. This statement is consistent with the vast majority of conditions that have an underlying nonstructural injury. These include fibromyalgia, neuropathies, neuralgias, neuromuscular dysfunction, and most painful conditions.

Since some complex conditions are due to multiple nonbeneficial instinctual responses, treatment will need to involve identifying and removing all of them. This process is similar to peeling off the layers of an onion. A better way to understand this concept is through the following example.

Imagine a glass filled with sand in the bottom one third and with water in the upper two thirds. Now imagine that the sand represents the instinctual responses that benefit you and the water represents the instinctual responses that are responsible for your clinical dysfunction. The goal of treatment is to remove the nonbeneficial ones, or the water, so that only the sand or the responses that benefit you remain in the glass. Undergoing neuroreactive medical treatment is similar to simply pouring the water out of the glass without losing any of the sand. When you try to do this, you will find that your first attempt or treatment will result in most of the water being removed. This will be recognized by the dramatic clinical improvement you will experience as a result of a single treatment since you will improve by the percentage of water that was removed. The classic example of this approach is overcoming the immobility due to stroke. Further treatment that removes more of the water or nonbeneficial instinctual responses will result in further clinical improvement.

# CHAPTER 4

*Overcoming The Way Others View Your Chronic*
*Nonstructural Injury*

## The inseparable disability

Logically, things should be just great if you actually got better and recovered from a significant injury. I initially thought that this was true, but it is not. This was brought to my attention by someone who I had successfully treated two weeks earlier. This patient said that she had been having problems since I had treated her. She had experienced restoration of normal movement, sensation, and function of her arm, as well as the elimination of disabling neuralgias. I inquired if her arm continued to be without pain and had normal sensation, and she said yes. I then asked if she had normal movement and function, and she again replied yes. So what was wrong?

She related that she went home and showed her family and friends that she got better, but they did not believe it. At a family get-together, she demonstrated that she was indeed fully functional and better. One would have thought that this would be a very happy and joyous occasion, but this is not what occurred. Instead of being happy that she had overcome her disabling pain, her family had the opposite reaction. They were upset with her. They also claimed that she had been faking her illness for the past several years. She was greatly distressed that her family and close friends thought that she faked her illness or derived some benefit from pretending to be disabled. Her family's reaction deeply hurt this patient.

This is a common human reaction to a person who was able to overcome disability through a different treatment that is not comprehended or commonly understood to be possible.

**When a severe long term disability is present, people learn to accept the person as well as the person's disability. The person and disability become inseparable in the minds of others.**

A change has to take place in order for others to disassociate the disability from the person. This transformation is necessary so that others can recognize the successfully treated patient as a different, newly functional individual. Those who routinely interact with a formerly disabled individual have to undergo change as well. They have to reorient their brains to react to this person in a different and more positive way. They also have to learn to treat him or her as a fully functional individual.

### Gaining Acceptance From The Brain Of Others Who Cannot Adjust

It can take time for the mind to reassess and reorient itself to properly behave and interact with such individuals. Many people's brains are slightly rigid or resistant to sudden change. What is needed to facilitate the process of conscious change is the understanding of how the affected person overcame his or her dysfunction. This must occur in order for the recovered patient to be accepted by those, who only knew him or her as someone who was different.

Ordinary people understand this type of transformation in traditional medical terms that are narrow and limited. The reason that someone was able overcome a disability is usually understood and socially accepted if one of the following scenarios occur. The first scenario is that an individual made a recovery after undergoing a new treatment or surgery. The anticipated reaction is the acceptance and the acknowledgment that, "If I ever experienced a similar problem, I would seek that doctor and undergo the same treatment." The second scenario is that a new medication was used to produce a miraculous cure. This explanation is appreciated by ordinary people. They will often inquire, "What is the name of the medication?" "How much did it cost and where can I get some?"

It is difficult for people to accept new treatments that they have neither experienced nor heard of. This is especially true if it is simple, does not involve any procedures, and can be performed in a single visit. One way to counteract this resistance is through awareness that a potential cure actually exists.

## Dysfunctional Interpersonal Relationships

Another outcome of treatment of a nonbeneficial instinctual response may include the disruption of a relationship in which the disability plays a central role. Relationships between two people are the sum of the interactions that occur between them. These anticipated and understood interactions allow two individuals to get along so that their relationship continues to be harmonious. The ability to get along may also be heavily strained by children, relatives, or friends. Fortunately, children are usually very receptive and happy when their parent is able to recover from an injury. Children see their moms and dads as loving providers of care and do not naturally view themselves as the ones who are supposed to be the caregiver.

A potential threat to a relationship may occur when one member is not able to handle their partner changing or recovering from an injury, even though it is for the better. This is even more of an issue if the relationship was not going well to begin with. It is disturbing that many people do not want their significant other to change, improve, or recover. These insecure individuals have their own issues to deal with including fear and jealousy. Frequently, there are underlying control issues and feelings of inadequacy regarding being with a partner who has overcome a serious disability. Some spouses feel that once their role as caregivers is over, they will no longer be needed. The thought of being outsourced, as well as the loss of purpose, sets forth a tidal wave of emotions and controlling behavior that needs to be dealt with immediately.

Frequently, these feelings surface when one partner has to deal with a perception that other same sex individuals may find someone who overcame his or her disability more attractive and desirable. Failure to deal with the troubled spouse may cause these behaviors to worsen to the point where dissolution of the relationship and separation occur. When I ask my patients why separation occurs, the usual answer is, "My former spouse became overly controlling, jealous, and unable to accept my recovery." Other common answers include, "He should have been happy that I underwent a change," and "If he really loved me, he would have wanted me to get better and feel better."

Another outcome of successful treatment may be a further deterioration of an already troubled relationship. Some people are unable to leave a relationship for a number of reasons, including their own insecurity, lack of financial independence, or issues concerning children. A frequent issue is that if things were not good before one partner recovered from a disability, then they may worsen after recovery. These individuals fear the potential of being treated even worse including experiencing increased abuse. One area of potential abuse frequently brought up is intimacy. In a relationship, some couples experience closeness and intimacy, while others do not. Intimacy can also be prevented by placing mutually agreed upon barriers. These provide an excuse so that the couple does not have to deal with deeper issues. These deeper underlying problems are the real issues why intimacy is not occurring. It is not important to elaborate on the deeper issues because couples who have them know quite well exactly what they are. It is important to note that a person's injury or ongoing symptoms is frequently one such barrier. The following case helps demonstrate this point.

Sophia is a thirty-two year old who came to my practice while visiting from Florida. She had previously experienced a water skiing accident in which she hit a large object. This had left her with a loss of sensation or numbness over her entire left leg as well as the inability to rotate her hip bone and upper leg in an outward direction. This injury persisted for three years and was not responsive to traditional medical treatment, including occupational and physical therapy.

When I saw her, I recognized her symptoms as being consistent with a nonstructural brain injury characterized by the nonbeneficial instinctual responses of hypersensitivity, numbness, and the loss of movement secondary to excruciating pain.  Sophia's brain was refusing to allow her to fully recover.  I was able to correct Sophia's nonstructural injury so that she was a completely different person than the one who had entered my office.  Sophia was able to feel normal sensation once again. Her pain had vanished, and she had full range of mobility of her leg.  She left my office very happy with the understanding that she could comfortably move her leg and even enjoy intimate relations.

What she did not tell me earlier was that her relationship was already deeply strained and that the mutually agreed upon barrier to intimacy was her injury. I followed up with her a few days later and she related the following.  She told me that although she feels perfectly fine, she had not even told her husband. I asked her why. She said that if he knew that she had recovered from her injury, then he would expect that they would be able to be intimate once again. She did not want that to occur.  Her painful leg was a mutually agreed upon barrier in the relationship and the only thing that kept him away.  The nonstructural brain injury that occurred due to an accidental trauma had formed a mutually agreed upon barrier to intimacy. This response was beneficial to her and allowed her to survive her dysfunctional and troubled relationship.

## The Superhero Analogy

This type of behavior is similar to the way our favorite dysfunctional superhero behaves. Our favorite superheroes appear to be disabled when they are around others.  They blend into the background so that they are not noticed, and when others are not around, they are able to act in a manner not characteristic of the physically injured. One similarity between a superhero and a person in a troubled relationship who overcame a nonstructural brain injury is that both individuals are never accepted when their actual identity is revealed. The result is that both go to great lengths to hide their powers in order to lead a more peaceful existence. This comparison can also lead to speculative thinking about the personal preferences and life experiences of those who write superhero scripts for Hollywood.

This chapter serves as a reminder that it is not enough to simply overcome the effects of a brain that refuses to allow itself to heal. In order to journey on the road to recovery, you need to avoid the potential potholes by effectively dealing with other individuals whose brains refuse to accept your ability to improve and get better.

# PART TWO

*Applying A Neuroreactive Approach To Overcome A Brain That Prevents Itself From Recovering*

**"Can this form of medical treatment really allow me to improve the way I feel and function?"**

The rest of this book will examine the way neuroreactive medicine addresses the specific illnesses, injuries, and dysfunctions that your brain may suffer from. You will gain valuable insight into how your mind functions as well as how neuroreactive medicine can be successfully applied. The previously discussed principles and pathways will be adjusted and modified to demonstrate that each topic or illness presented is really a similar example of the way the brain refuses to allow itself to get better. By recognizing how the brain can become injured and develop the instinctual responses that do not benefit your well being, you will realize that treatment is possible using a neuroreactive approach.

**The treatment for all of the individual cases and conditions examined in this book is similar. It is based on how the brain clinically functions. Treatment is accomplished through the following steps:**

**1. Recognizing that a nonstructural injury is present because you cannot treat what you are unable to recognize as being present.**

**2. Bypassing the critical conscious thought process (using any method).**

**3. Establishing effective communication with the subconscious thought process where the nonstructural brain injury is located.**

**4. Identifying and eliminating the nonstructural injury that produced an individual's nonbeneficial instinctual responses.**

**5. Retraining the brain to instinctually respond in a beneficial manner similar to the way it did prior to experiencing the injury.**

* * *

**See It For Yourself**

Since seeing is believing, I would like to provide you with the opportunity to see for yourself how neuroreactive treatment can deeply affect many individuals' lives and enable them to improve. They are actual people who have been treated and who were kind enough to grant the use of their testimonials. You will be amazed to see how they are dramatically improved and well again after just a single treatment. These altruistic individuals have allowed the use of their videos so that others who suffer from the same symptoms, disease, or dysfunction can see that an innovative and effective approach is available. They are not paid actors; they are ordinary people, just like yourself.

You may find these videos on the website **<Amazingtreatment. com>** or on the Internet at **youtube.com** when you search under the title **Dr. Richard G. Herman.**

Finally, it is worthy to note that the cases presented in this book illustrate what is medically achievable when you apply the principles of neuroreactive medicine to the illness or injury from which you suffer. They are based on actual individuals encountered in clinical practice. Since there are very few truly unique presentations of a given illness or disease process, it is obvious that there are many other people who suffer from the same symptoms and dysfunctions that you suffer from. That is why aspects of their stories will seem familiar to you. In order to respect the subjects, their names and identifying details have been altered. It is also worthy to note that the individuals videotaped on the web site are not the patients whose stories are portrayed in this book. Any attempt to connect a case presented in this book or on the web site with an individual that you know of will not be accurate.

# CHAPTER 5

*The Brain That Refused To Overcome Acute and Chronic Illness*

Illnesses can affect individuals in different ways. What we fail to realize is that a significant percentage of the conditions that affect us are directly due to the way our brain prevents itself from recovering. Despite the different ways diseases present, the nonstructural brain consistently responds in the same way.

This chapter explores how the brain responds to different illnesses that prevent it from allowing itself to get better. These challenges include those disease processes that are acute or self limiting and those that are chronic or ongoing.

## Responding to Illness

If you have to contract an illness, it will hopefully be self-limiting. These are the ones that you experience and then completely forget about because they have no long lasting effects on your well being. Your body's immune system effectively does its job to heal you so you are able to function at full capacity once more. Examples include colds, infections, and minor musculoskeletal injuries. The fact that you do not have any significant long-term dysfunction means that you did not develop any nonstructural brain injuries that needed to be overcome. An additional beneficial response subconsciously occurs so that you learn and develop appropriate instinctual reactions that help you adapt and learn to deal with the same or similar illnesses in the future.

Two neuroreactive principles that need to be kept in mind are the following:

**The faster that you can fully overcome an illness, the less likely that you may experience ongoing dysfunction by developing a nonstructural injury.**

Another principle includes the following observation.

**The ongoing symptoms due to a nonstructural injury will not go away until it is addressed and treated.**

Failure to recognize these principles frequently results in under treatment because the brain is refusing to allow itself to get better. People who experience this type of injury know their symptoms are real and interfere with their ability to function on a daily basis. They will go to great lengths to seek treatment that is usually limited to the structural diagnosis and its accompanying chronic symptoms. Unfortunately, these people do not get better because treatment is not directed at the underlying cause.

Some illnesses are present for a very limited time period, yet the symptoms remain long after it has vanished. One reason is that the illness has also affected the subconscious thought process through the production of a nonstructural brain injury.

**When this occurs, the nonstructural brain is continually and instinctually responding incorrectly to a perceived illness that doesn't presently exist.**

This is a common presentation in clinical practice. People continue to experience significant pain and dysfunction long after the illness has gone away. The only thing that actually remains of the illness is the injury to the subconscious thought process that is producing the ongoing nonbeneficial instinctual response.

### Trigeminal Neuralgia

This type of response was seen in a person who had a severe case of adult chicken pox.  He had developed deep skin lesions, severe itching, and a burning sensation on the right cheek. After the chicken pox had resolved, the burning, itching sensation persisted and was aggravated by heat, including excessive sun exposure. The patient saw several clinicians, including specialists in otolaryngology and neurology. He was informed that his symptoms were the result of a trigeminal nerve injury (trigeminal neuralgia) due to his prior infection with chicken pox. He was told that the chicken pox lesions located just above the trigeminal nerve had injured this nerve, causing it to react in a way that produced his symptoms. He had tried traditional medical treatments, including creams and pills that failed to help. Eventually, he was told that nothing more could be done. His daily symptoms continued to persist for several years.

Individuals diagnosed with trigeminal neuralgia experience symptoms due to a structural injury involving the trigeminal nerve or fifth cranial nerve. Many times the exact causes of this injury are unknown. These symptoms vary in severity and intensity and are characterized by pain sensations occurring hundreds of times each day. Some have described their pain as shock like, stabbing, shooting, or twisting. Pain can also be precipitated by everyday actions, such as chewing, talking, brushing teeth, or even touching a certain spot on the face. Treatment for this condition addresses the structural nerve injury, including time, medication, nerve blocks, acupuncture, or even dental surgery.

Some patients have even considered undergoing gamma beam irradiation to the trigeminal nerve. If a purely structural injury to the trigeminal nerve is present, most patients would get better using medical treatment targeting the trigeminal nerve. Since many do not improve, it is appropriate to consider that a nonstructural injury may be contributing to the symptoms of trigeminal neuralgia. If this were indeed the case, then it would be reasonable to expect that the symptoms of trigeminal neuralgia would resolve after treatment.

When a nonstructural injury is present, effective treatment is directed at the subconscious mind or the source and not at the distal site where the symptoms occur. This form of injury was consistent with this individual's symptoms. His nonstructural brain was unable to separate the symptoms due to severe irritation of the trigeminal nerve versus chicken pox because of the lesions close proximity to the trigeminal nerve. The result was the development of a nonstructural injury characterized by a nonbeneficial instinctual response that included a persistent burning and itching sensation on the right cheek. These symptoms were present long after the illness that produced them had resolved. Once this injury was recognized, it was easily treated. Clearly, many cases of trigeminal neuralgia are not entirely due to an ongoing structural injury. A neuroreactive medical approach can provide great benefit to those who continue to suffer when their brains refuse to allow them to get better.

### Responding To Chronic Illness

Illnesses are considered chronic when the underlying disease cannot be eliminated. Management attempts to prevent further deterioration as well as control any symptoms that may be present. From a neuroreactive standpoint, the following principles may apply.

**The longer a disease persists, the greater the likelihood that you may experience ongoing dysfunction secondary to the development of a nonstructural injury.**

**The greater the extent of the symptoms and ongoing severity of an illness, the greater the probability that you will experience an ongoing nonstructural injury.**

**The greater the possibility that you are unable to consciously deal with a chronic illness, the more likely a subconscious nonstructural injury in the form of a nonbeneficial instinctual reaction will occur.**

The nonstructural brain only remains in control for a certain period of time before experiencing injury from chronic illness. When this occurs, there are then two locations of ongoing injury. The first is the structural area on the body that is affected. The second is the additional dysfunction due to the nonbeneficial instinctual reactions resulting from the disease's effect on the nonstructural brain. These nonbeneficial instinctual reactions will persist if the chronic illness remains stable. They may even worsen as the disease progresses.

## Multiple Sclerosis

Tim came to see me with the diagnosis of multiple sclerosis for the past ten years. Multiple sclerosis is a chronic inflammatory disease that affects the central nervous system. Those who deal with this illness frequently fail to consider that a nonstructural brain injury also contributes to this illness's ongoing symptomatology.

Many who are diagnosed with early multiple sclerosis experience periods of symptomatic relapse as well as periods of relative remittance that can occur over many years. Treatment involves the use of medication aimed at preventing progression, relapse, and addressing the symptoms that are present. Affected individuals may display symptoms that include fatigue, spasticity, motor weakness, pain, ataxia, pressure, and altered sensitivity.

Tim experienced many of the symptoms listed above and had significant lesions noted on his imaging studies. He was particularly burdened by fatigue, hypersensitivity to touch, pins and needles sensations, and stabbing leg pain. These were not relieved by traditional medical treatment.

The first consideration is that these symptoms are due to the multiple sclerosis producing an ongoing structural injury. If this is the case, then the symptoms should persist despite being neuroreactively treated. After all, the structural disease producing the symptoms would still be present and unchanged by the treatment. This is consistent with the following principle.

**Neuroreactive treatment only treats the nonstructural component of a given condition and has no effect on any actual structural disease that is present.**

The other consideration is to determine if the multiple sclerosis had affected the nonstructural brain to produce a nonbeneficial instinctual reaction that contributed to the ongoing pain and suffering. If this is the case, it would explain why the ongoing hypersensitivity to touch, pins and needles sensations, and pain in his legs were not relieved by traditional medical treatment. Tim overcame his dysfunction through neuroreactive treatment. Two years later he continued to be pain free.

Multiple sclerosis is an ongoing disease whose symptoms appear receptive to neuroreactive treatment, especially in the early stages. In later stage disease, there is a much larger percentage of permanent structural musculoskeletal dysfunction that would not be receptive to this approach. You cannot eliminate the multiple sclerosis since it is a disease that progressively produces physical structural changes. You can only remove the nonbeneficial instinctual responses that contribute to the dysfunction an individual with multiple sclerosis may experience. While the results of treatment can provide significant symptom relief, the disease may continue to slowly progress and reinjure the subconscious brain; therefore, a similar or different presentation of symptoms may occur in the future. It is also important to recognize that multiple sclerosis has not been linked with a specific preventable behavioral cause that can be avoided to prevent progression or future flare-ups. This is in contrast to other chronic illnesses such as uncontrolled diabetes that can immediately increase the possibility of reinjury of the subconscious mind.

### Neuroreactive Reinjury

This observation is consistent with the following principles.

**Once a chronic disease is controlled by medical treatment and any nonstructural injuries are addressed, no further nonstructural symptoms are expected to occur unless the subconscious brain is reinjured.**

**The more difficult it is to maintain control due to a chronic illness, the more likely reinjury will occur.**

I encourage patients who suffer from multiple sclerosis to follow their neurologist's recommended medication protocol in order to keep the disease inactive and to prevent further progression. Neuro-reactive treatment is additionally recommended to remove the nonbeneficial instinctual responses that contribute to the patient's symptoms. This protocol appears to work significantly better than either approach used individually. It seems to offer a better long term result of remaining unaffected by the symptoms that previously were present. This combined approach also prevents under treatment when considerable improvement is possible.

### Fibromyalgia

Fibromyalgia is a syndrome in which patients suffer from chronic, diffuse pain over their entire body. Individuals routinely experience chronic fatigue, insomnia, and multiple tender trigger points that are present at the points of muscle insertion. Many complain of severe pressure involving their arms and legs, causing sensations of bruising and soreness. The statement, "I ache all over, especially if you squeeze me," is not uncommon.

A typical case is that of a patient named Rachel who wanted me to treat her fibromyalgia. It had been constantly present for at least twenty years. Every muscle of her body was intensely achy to touch so that she felt the constant sensation of pressure. She had seen multiple specialists and tried numerous treatments, all of which came up short. She continued to feel discomfort from soreness, pressure, and multiple painful trigger points. Most of all, she experienced a hurting sensation as if someone were constantly squeezing all of her muscles. Like so many others, Rachel had tried several other unsuccessful medical treatments and was skeptical of the possibility of improvement. She initially did not believe me when I casually told her that improvement could occur in just a single visit. I told her that her pain would be gone and that she would be able to squeeze herself as hard as she wanted to without feeling any soreness, achiness, or pressure. I based these comments on the clinical success that I have had treating many other patients using a neuroreactive medical approach. Fibromyalgia appears to have a significant component of nonstructural injury expressed as ongoing nonbeneficial instinctual reactions. It appears that the brain of many individuals with fibromyalgia refuses to allow these people to overcome their symptoms and get better. Treatment is simple. Once these reactions are removed, the symptoms go away and are not expected to return. After treatment, all of Rachel's symptoms disappeared and did not return, as I confirmed via a follow up visit at a later date.

### The Squeeze Test

Although the exact cause of fibromyalgia is not known, it is not necessary to determine the reason for the dysfunction in order to provide effective relief. I have found that a simple squeeze test can help predict successful treatment. When examining an individual who claims to suffer from fibromyalgia, it is important to determine if there are any clinical symptoms present. Although many individuals claim this diagnosis, not all of them actually have this diagnosis. A simple squeeze test over the muscles in the arms and legs will help identify those who will respond favorably to treatment. If the patient exhibits pain, discomfort, hypersensitivity, or achy pressure, even with light touch, we should suspect that a very treatable nonstructural component is present.

### Sjogren's Syndrome, Sclerodactyly, and Grip Dysfunction

Many illnesses appear to have a significant nonstructural component that once recognized can be addressed. These include diseases that have limited treatment options. Sjogren's syndrome is one of them. This syndrome is a chronic inflammatory disorder that frequently affects women in their middle ages. Dryness of the mouth, eyes, and mucous membranes characterize this syndrome. For Mary, this syndrome meant constant dryness and discomfort. Mary took all of her prescribed medications and supplemented her inability to produce saliva by taking frequent sips of water and chewing gum.

These measures failed to provide any meaningful relief. She also experienced diffuse fibrosis of her hands or sclerodactyly. This made it difficult to close her hands or make a fist, which resulted in a very weak grip. Mary was referred to my practice by a friend who thought that I could help her. Using the principles outlined in this book, Mary achieved the most remarkable improvement. She is now able to have normal production of saliva, and the dryness that affected her eyes has vanished. She is also amazed that she is able to fully move her fingers once more and that her grip is strong and firm. One year later, Mary still felt improved and quite pleased that she underwent treatment.

# CHAPTER 6

*The Diabetic Brain*

Our brains are very susceptible to the effects of diabetes. This chapter will redefine the way this disease is traditionally viewed through understanding the functioning of the diabetic brain that refuses to allow itself to get better. You will learn how it is possible to overcome the brain's ability to instinctively feel pain when you check your blood sugar or administer insulin. You will also discover how the symptoms of diabetic neuropathy are intimately related to the way the brain instinctually responds and is affected by diabetes. This knowledge will reveal that the symptoms of neuropathy can be eliminated by addressing the underlying nonstructural injury to the diabetic brain.

**How We Perceive Pain**

When we think about diabetes, we think about people monitoring their blood sugar levels by sticking their finger with a lancet. A lancet is a short, sharp needle used to obtain a drop of blood. When an abnormal elevated blood sugar reading is obtained, it is treated by administering a shot filled with insulin.

**Understanding How The Brain Senses Pain From A Needle Stick**

The process is initiated when a sharp needle enters the skin and sends a signal from this distal site to the nonstructural brain. This signal reaches and challenges the nonstructural brain to respond to this injury so that a loss of control can be avoided. The nonstructural brain accepts this signal and responds by interpreting the needle stick as pain. The nonstructural brain is able to maintain control through acknowledging the needle stick injury. This leads to the symptoms of acute pain at the site of the needle stick, ongoing soreness, and tenderness to the touch. It also imprints and reinforces the subconscious memory to instinctively respond similarly to any further needle sticks. This explanation is consistent with the belief that pain can be initiated by sticking your finger with a lancet or administering insulin via a shot.

### An Experiment That Challenges Our Perceptions Of Pain

A series of experiments were conducted to challenge our perceptions concerning pain. The initial goal was to prove that a person would be expected to feel pain as a result of a needle stick injury. Ten random people had their blood drawn and were questioned if they felt pain at the needle injury site. All ten responded that they did. This simple experiment confirms the obvious conclusion that if you are stuck with a needle, you should feel pain in response to the needle stick. These results are consistent with the discomfort you felt the last time you accidentally stuck yourself with a sharp object or a needle.

What if it were possible to challenge these results and arrive at a completely different conclusion. This new hypothesis would state that you would not feel pain when stuck with a needle. If this statement was found to be true, it would challenge our perception of how the brain functions. To prove this assumption, we used two random groups of ten individuals who needed to get their blood drawn. The first group of ten individuals simply had their blood drawn and were asked if they felt pain at the needle injury site. The second group underwent the same blood draw five minutes after listening to a brief neuroreactive discussion. The results were remarkably the opposite for each group. Members of the first group that simply underwent a blood draw all felt pain at the needle injury site. Participants in the other group that received a discussion prior to the needle draw all reported that they did not feel any pain at the needle injury site.

Now imagine if I touched you with the same sharp needle and you did not feel any pain. What if I took this test a step further and touched you with the same needle several times in multiple places, including your forehead and gums, and you still reported that you did not feel anything. If this was possible, you would question how this could occur because you know that when you are stuck with a needle you are supposed to feel pain.

The obvious conclusion is that something happened to the subconscious thought process in those individuals who listened to the neuroreactive discussion. Since this is possible, we are obligated to rethink the way we are programmed to respond to pain. From the above experiment, we are led to consider the following principles:

**We only experience pain when the brain allows us to feel pain.**

**When the brain does not allow us to feel pain, we do not experience pain.**

* * *

### A New Understanding Of How The Diabetic Brain Senses Pain From A Needle Stick

The traditional way to trigger a painful response starts with the act of monitoring your blood sugar by sticking your finger with a lancet or administering insulin. When the sharp needle enters the skin, it sends a signal from this distal site to the nonstructural brain. This signal challenges the nonstructural brain to respond to this injury so that a loss of control can be avoided. The nonstructural brain is able to stay in control because it has been enabled to instinctually respond in a different, more beneficial manner. It does not accept this signal of injury and does not interpret the needle stick as pain. This results in <u>not</u> experiencing the symptoms of acute pain at the site of the needle stick, ongoing soreness, or tenderness to the touch.

This pathway is consistent with my findings in clinical practice. People only experience pain when the brain allows them to feel pain. This is reflected in the following principle.

**We behave according to the way we instinctually respond.**

If it is possible that you can instinctually respond to experience pain that is nonbeneficial to your well being, then it must also be possible to instinctually respond in a beneficial manner not to feel the same pain or discomfort.

**The clinical significance is that diabetics can find it completely unnecessary to feel pain when they stick themselves to monitor their blood sugar or administer a shot of insulin.**

It is not a difficult thing to clinically achieve. Just imagine what a profound positive effect the ability not to feel pain due to needle sticks would have on a diabetic. You can make the unpleasant and uncomfortable act of getting stuck with a needle into one that leads to no pain or discomfort. Pain is a significant reason why many diabetics do not keep good control of their blood sugars. They do not want to feel pain when they are stuck. This discovery could have a significant impact on many people's willingness to maintain better glycemic control as well as avoid the complications that occur due to noncompliance.

An understanding of the brain's contribution to the perception of pain is seen in the following principle.

**Many conditions including pain can be improved when treatment addresses the instinctual reactions of the subconscious mind and does not solely focus on the distal site where the pain is felt.**

This principle can be applied to a significant number of chronic illnesses, including diabetic neuropathy.

## Diabetic Neuropathy

I see many individuals who suffer from the effects of chronic diabetes, which is a disease that I tell my patients that they are too sweet for themselves. They face numerous challenges including the ability to maintain proper control of their blood sugars. When their disease worsens, neuropathy can occur over time. For many, diabetic neuropathy means living without normal sensitivity to touch that nondiabetics take for granted. Diabetics have described this as having fingers and toes that they cannot feel are even there. This is associated with muscle cramps, hot and cold episodes, numbness, lack of feeling, and loss of fine motor skills. Others experience sensations of pins and needles, tingling, and the inability to recognize when an extremity is bleeding or bruised. Diabetic neuropathy is referred to as a chronic disease in which the symptoms cannot usually be overcome. Even though many people try different treatments and medications, the symptoms of the neuropathy continue to affect them negatively every waking minute of their day. The option given to most people is simply putting up with the symptoms of the neuropathy as best they can.

Most of the treatments that are prescribed are aimed at making diabetic neuropathy livable. They are usually directed at the extremities and commonly include supportive devices, heat, massage, and medication. These treatments are not exceedingly effective because they are only targeting a location of the body that may not be completely responsible for producing a diabetic's symptoms. One area of the body that may be responsible includes a brain that refuses to allow itself to get better. This is present when diabetes adversely affects the brain to produce a nonstructural injury in addition to the peripheral injury. This is understood by examining the relationship between diabetic neuropathy and the way that nonstructural brain injury affects your symptoms.

Diabetic neuropathy is usually not present when people initially develop diabetes. Most people simply don't go from developing diabetes to immediately experiencing the symptoms of neuropathy. Something usually has to happen before they develop the neuropathy.

Neuropathy frequently develops over time when a person's diabetes is not tightly controlled through proper diet, exercise, appropriate body weight, healthy lifestyle changes, strict glycemic control, and aggressive management of any other chronic diseases or illnesses. Those suffering from diabetic neuropathy are frequently losing their battle with other chronic illnesses in addition to their ongoing poor glycemic control. Their attention and focus is centered on the location where they perceive that their neuropathy is present. I rarely see anyone who has not tried at least several different medications and treatments, all of which failed to provide the desired result.

When diabetes is present, it is not only producing symptoms, injury, and dysfunction peripherally on the body or at the site where it hurts. It is also affecting the nonstructural portion of the brain located in the subconscious mind.

### How Diabetic Neuropathy Can Produce A Nonstructural Brain Injury

Ongoing poorly controlled diabetes

Diabetes eventually affects and potentially injures the body, including the nerves located in the distal arms and legs

This injury signals and challenges the nonstructural brain to respond to the injury that these nerves are experiencing so that a temporary state of loss of control occurs in the subconscious mind. This results in

↓

Nonstructural brain confusion

This reflects the brain's ability to respond to and overcome the loss of control due to the symptoms or dysfunction caused by the diabetes affecting the nervous system in the arms and legs.

↓← The effects of medical treatment include the impact

↓ of medication, proper diet,

↓ weight loss, strict glycemic control,

↓ healthy lifestyle changes, as well as treatment for other

↓ chronic illnesses.

↓

Despite treatment, the subconscious, nonstructural brain is unable to completely resolve the ongoing loss of control from the chronic and frequently uncontrolled diabetes.

↓

Instinctual imprinting occurs over time

This results in some portions of the subconscious, nonstructural brain remaining in control and being unaffected by the diabetes.

Other portions of the subconscious, nonstructural brain are now over-ridden or reprogrammed by the process of instinctual imprinting. This leads to the formation of a…

↓

Nonstructural brain injury

A nonstructural brain injury occurs due to the inability of the subconscious, nonstructural brain to resolve the loss of control, including the subsequent negative instinctual imprinting that occurred.

↓

The result of this type of injury is that a nonbeneficial instinctual response is formed. From this point on, the portion of the subconscious mind that was injured will respond in an inappropriate way.

This type of injury may be clinically recognizable by the symptoms of neuropathy. These nonbeneficial changes significantly contribute as a percentage to a person's overall diabetic neuropathy.

Once a nonstructural brain injury or nonbeneficial instinctual response is recognized, it can be treated successfully. Thus, the percentage that the nonbeneficial instinctual response contributed to a person's overall neuropathy can be eliminated. Many times this results in significant and noticeable clinical improvement.

The symptoms of neuropathy should not return unless the subconscious mind is reinjured. This may result from poor glycemic control, unhealthy lifestyle changes, and/or failure to treat other chronic illnesses that are present.

\*\*\*

If the symptoms of a nonstructural injury relating to diabetic neuropathy can be effectively treated, then what can be done to ensure that they do not return? This question is clinically appreciated using the following analogy.

### A Penny Jar Analogy

Remember a time in your childhood when you placed a very dark brown penny in a jar and then poured various liquids into the jar to see what happened to the penny? Imagine that the penny represents your nerves and the various fluids correspond to the different environments that your nerves are exposed to. Now try to visualize what this would look like in a normal individual.

In a normal individual, the fluid in the jar can be compared to water so that the very dark brown penny would be completely unaffected by the water. This is similar to people who have good control of their blood sugars. As long as a diabetic's blood sugars remain in a normal range, there is little risk that his or her nerves will be affected or this person will develop neuropathy.

In the case of one who suffers from diabetic neuropathy, you can compare the fluid in the jar to the highly acidic fluid found in a can of soda. You know what happens to a dark brown penny that is placed inside of a jar filled with soda. The harsh acidic liquid starts to eat away at the penny. Over time, the penny starts to look more dysfunctional. The injury to the penny is analogous to a diabetic neuropathy that is produced from actual nerve injury as well as the additional injury sustained by the nonstructural brain.

A diabetic can prevent further neurologic injury by removing the harsh environment and replacing it with a fluid that prevents further damage. This is accomplished by a combination of corrective measures, including weight loss, dietary control, healthy lifestyle changes, and treatment of other present chronic illnesses. Excellent ongoing glycemic control is also required.

When this change occurs, the uncontrolled diabetes, or the reason that produced the nonstructural brain injury, has stopped negatively affecting this person, but the individual continues to experience the symptoms of diabetic neuropathy. The traditional way of viewing this disease is that the symptoms caused by the damaged nerves occurring in the extremities will persist. These symptoms may possibly improve with medication but will recur as soon as the medication wears off. The ability to treat individuals is greatly enhanced by understanding diabetic neuropathy as not just a disease that affects the peripheral nerves but one that also affects the nonstructural brain by producing nonbeneficial instinctual responses.

### Treatment Considerations

When a long-term nonstructural brain injury is present, effective treatment is directed at the source of the injury and not necessarily at the distal site where the symptoms are present. This area of injury is located in the subconscious mind. In order to treat the subconscious mind, you have to be able to bypass the conscious thought process that prevents access to it. This form of therapy can eliminate the symptoms of nonstructural diabetic neuropathy. Once these symptoms are resolved, they should not return unless the nonstructural brain is subjected to a similar loss of control. This can occur if a person does not maintain proper control of the illness that produced the symptoms initially or is reinjured as a result of another chronic illness.

### An Example Of The Diabetic Brain That Allowed Itself To Get Better

Kathy has had diabetes for several years. Due to her busy lifestyle, she did not find it important to look after herself. Her priorities led her on a different path that resulted in poor compliance with both her diet and her ability to maintain proper blood sugars. She was able to live with her diabetes because it was essentially a disease on paper and did not physically affect her. She was a self described, "If it isn't broken, then don't fix it," type of person. Over time, she experienced considerable weight gain, making it increasingly difficult to control her blood sugars. She was placed on medication, and when this failed to help her, she graduated to insulin shots.

She eventually started experiencing symptoms of diabetic neuropathy. These included muscle cramps, pins and needles sensations, tingling, and numbness. An interesting thing suddenly occurred. She finally woke up and started to take her disease seriously. She had realized that something was broken that desperately needed to be fixed. So she set about fixing it by taking her diet seriously and losing a considerable amount of weight. She also found that as she lost weight, she only required a very low dose of an oral medication to control her blood sugars.

Although her control of her diabetes took a dramatic turn for the better, she still experienced ongoing symptoms due to the neuropathy. This was initially treated with traditional medication that caused her to feel tired and have persistent stomach irritation. Kathy's ongoing symptoms sounded similar to many patients that I have helped in the past. Kathy's diabetes had not only affected the peripheral nerves in her extremities, but had also adversely affected the way her nonstructural brain responded to the injury. This led to the formation of a nonstructural brain injury characterized by ongoing nonbeneficial instinctual responses. When treatment was directed at the source of the injury, eighty-five percent of Kathy's neuropathy resolved. The remaining fifteen percent of her symptoms were due to an actual structural neurological lesion. Once these symptoms are resolved, they should not be expected to return unless the nonstructural brain is subjected to a similar loss of control in the future. This can occur if a person does not maintain proper control of the illness that produced the symptoms initially. Nine months later, Kathy continued to maintain excellent control of her diabetes and did not experience any recurrence of her symptoms.

**Neuroreactive Reinjury**

Beth Ann had suffered from insulin dependent diabetes for well over ten years. Her disease had progressed to the point where even medication could not remove the diabetic neuropathy that included sensations of pins and needles, burning pain, and numbness. Once her nonstructural injury was identified and addressed, it became possible for her brain to function properly as it did in the distant past.

Beth Ann was reinterviewed seven weeks later. She was quite happy with the noticeable changes that took place. These included the elimination of the majority of her symptoms that included the sensation of pins and needles, burning pain, and numbness. She reported that she once again had the ability to feel her feet as well as her toes moving in her shoes. She also was able to feel objects with her fingers, even with her eyes closed. Beth Ann still reported that there was a small component of numbness attributable to an actual structural injury caused by the diabetic neuropathy.

Unfortunately, Beth Ann was not able to maintain a proper diet. Her blood sugars started to spiral out of control. One day they were high, and the next day they were even higher. Beth Ann also suffered from other chronic illnesses that included chronic pancreatitis, hypertension, and congestive heart failure. Four weeks later, she contracted an infection in her bloodstream that caused her to be hospitalized. Due to the severity of her illness, she required intubation and needed to be placed on a ventilator. After she was able to breathe on her own once more, she discovered that the symptoms of her diabetic neuropathy had recurred.

This case helps explain why the results of a treatment that appears overwhelmingly successful initially, seems to not last over time. The reason that Beth Ann's symptoms returned was not due to the initial treatment being unsuccessful. Her symptoms returned because her subconscious mind experienced a **neuroreactive reinjury** when it was unable to overcome a loss of control.

This form of reinjury is similar to the following scenario. Imagine you underwent a successful surgery to treat a knee injury. Six months later, you suddenly lose control of your balance, experience a fall, and reinjure the knee. Do you blame the original knee surgery as being unsuccessful? Of course not, because the knee's present dysfunction is due to a separate injury. Then who do we blame? We secretly blame ourselves for not being more careful to ensure that the benefits of our prior treatment will last and endure.

This example teaches us that individuals who are poorly controlled and who suffer from multiple additional chronic illnesses and comorbidities run a significant risk of reinjury and recurrence even after effective treatment. This is also true of the other chronic illnesses or injuries. Most individuals are expected to experience challenges as well as exacerbations or flare-ups over time. The only thing a physician can do is treat the patient as effectively as possible and then hope that the patient is able to make the correct decisions to maintain the benefits of that treatment to prevent reinjury.

### A Different Type Of Reinjury

There is also a different presentation of brain reinjury called **confusion reinjury**. This form occurs when there are two completely separate injuries affecting a given anatomic location, such as an arm or a leg. One of the injuries is a physical one, and the other is an unrelated nonstructural brain injury that is producing a separate nonbeneficial instinctual response at the site of the physical injury. An example includes the physical injury of chronic inflammation of the sole of the foot and the unrelated symptom of chronic numbness of the toes due to an adverse reaction to chemotherapy. The numbness due to the nonstructural injury was successfully eliminated by treatment. The problem occurs when the inflammation flares up. The numbness then returns and does not go away. When this situation is present, the brain becomes reinjured and responds in an abnormal fashion because it cannot overcome the confusion to distinguish between the actual physical injury and the memory of responding to the previously treated nonstructural injury. Individuals who experience this type of confusion reinjury can be successfully retreated. All that has to be done is to address this confusion to ensure that the subconscious mind understands that there are two separate injuries occurring. Once accomplished, the brain is able to respond to the actual physical injury without the reemergence of the nonstructural injury. In our example, the numbness goes away and does not return, even if a future episode of inflammation occurs.

In summary, this chapter is able to provide an innovative way to view the relationship between diabetes, diabetic nephropathy, and the development of nonstructural brain injury. Through the understanding that the brain can also be injured when it is unable to respond to the overwhelming loss of control it experiences as a result of poorly controlled diabetes, caregivers now have the opportunity to address and correct the nonstructural injuries that can occur.

# CHAPTER 7

### *The Brain That Refused To Heal Itself After A Stroke*

A new method of treatment exists that will enable many stroke victims to make significant clinical improvement not previously thought possible. Individuals who suffer from weakness or limited mobility are now able to regain normal movement. Through this treatment the brain regains control and returns to functioning the way it did prior to the stroke. You may ask if this is really possible. The answer is that it is possible and, surprisingly, it is not that difficult to achieve. This chapter will outline an innovative clinical understanding demonstrating how the nonstructural brain's ability to properly function is adversely affected by a stroke. Subsequently, you will learn that an effective treatment exists for the brain that refused to get better after experiencing a stroke.

### Stroke

A stroke, or cerebrovascular accident, is a devastating disease that affects many people every day. It occurs when a blood clot occludes one of the arteries in the brain. A stroke can prevent critical blood flow to portions of the brain responsible for the functioning of the nerves and muscles. When a portion of the brain is deprived of its blood supply, it sustains an injury which may result in actual tissue death as well subsequent neurologic and neuromuscular deficits.

These deficits include weakness or the inability to move your arms or legs, numbness, neuropathy, difficulties eating or speaking, visual disturbances, dizziness, and/or memory loss. Through medical intervention, time, and rehabilitation therapy, some people are able to improve their deficits. Many still have significant dysfunction preventing them from leading the life that they were supposed to have enjoyed. They are left to deal with the remaining dysfunction because they have been told that nothing more could be done. The end result is familiar to those who know of such people. These victims do not improve and time just goes on. What they fail to realize is that they also suffer from a brain that refuses to allow them to get better and overcome the dysfunction caused by their stroke.

### An Example Familiar To Those Who Have Suffered A Stroke

The following example will show what can be accomplished using a neuroreactive medical approach. This individual's doctor had heard of my special interest in helping stroke victims make great functional improvements after being told nothing more could be done.

Jim suffered a devastating cerebrovascular accident, or stroke, about two months after undergoing a successful abdominal surgery. The stroke involved the middle cerebral artery in his brain. When I saw Jim for the first time, it was visually apparent that he indeed had suffered from a major stroke in the distant past. I could plainly see that he suffered from limited mobility and that his left arm was still affected, appearing to be contracted at the elbow.

Twelve years earlier, Jim had a single major stroke that had left him with significant ongoing dysfunction. He told me that he still experiences the following dysfunctions and symptoms which may sound familiar to someone who has had a similar experience.

1. Limited mobility of his shoulder: He has not been able to raise his arm or reach above his shoulder for the last twelve years.

2. Limited mobility of his elbow to flex and extend: He cannot fully flex or extend his elbow. He can move it somewhat with considerable effort. Due to his inability to fully extend his elbow, it appears to be contracted or chronically bent. It appears that

his bicep muscle, located on the front part of the upper arm, is excessively pulling the elbow into flexion, and his triceps muscle, located on the back of the upper arm, is unable to counteract this flexion.

3. Weakness of his arm.

4. The inability to move the first and second fingers on his left hand.

5. Limited flexibility, movement, and strength of his third, fourth, and fifth finger.

6. Numbness of his face, particularly at the corner of the mouth.

Jim claimed that for the last twelve years he could not overcome these symptoms despite medication and seeing multiple specialists. He had participated in multiple years of physical therapy as well as a host of other promising treatments that did not improve his condition. For the last several years, he felt that he was just wasting his time and money with no improvement to show for it, so he became quite skeptical that any more improvement was possible. Jim also told me that the only reason he agreed to see me was that his doctor convinced him to. He said, "If it was anybody else but my doctor who told me to see you, I would not have come." Since he deeply respected his doctor, he came. I thanked him for coming and I told him I would do my best to live up to the kindness and faith that his doctor had shown in me.

In order to help Jim and the countless other individuals who suffer neuromuscular dysfunction from stroke, we need to rethink from a neuroreactive medical perspective how these limitations resulting from a stroke occurred. When we do so, it will lead to the understanding that many stroke victims are being under treated and that significant clinical improvement is readily achievable.

Using this patient's symptoms to show how this is possible, let us look at our innovative clinical pathway to see how it applies to stroke.

This outline will provide you with an understanding of how a stroke can injure the nonstructural brain to produce the neuromuscular dysfunction that you are unable to overcome.

### A Pathway That Changes The Way We View Injury Due To Stroke

An individual experiences a stroke or thromboembolic event to the brain

That produces symptoms, injury, and dysfunction in the structural brain

That signals and challenges the nonstructural brain to respond to the injury so that a temporary state of loss of control occurs in the subconscious mind. This results in

Nonstructural brain confusion

This reflects the brain's ability to respond to and overcome the loss of control due to the symptoms or dysfunction caused by the actual structural injury.

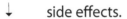 ← The effect of medical treatment including medications and its

↓    side effects.

Despite treatment, the subconscious, nonstructural brain is unable to completely resolve the loss of control.

Instinctual imprinting then occurs.

This results in some portions of the subconscious, nonstructural brain remaining in control and being unaffected by the stroke.

Other portions of the subconscious, nonstructural brain are now overridden or reprogrammed by the process of instinctual imprinting. This leads to the formation of a...

Nonstructural brain injury

A nonstructural brain injury occurs due to the inability of the subconscious, nonstructural brain to resolve the loss of control leading to the occurrence of subsequent negative instinctual imprinting.

The result of this type of injury is that a nonbeneficial instinctual response is formed. From this point on, the portion of the subconscious mind that was injured will respond in an inappropriate way.

↓

This type of injury may be clinically recognizable by the obvious neuromuscular dysfunction that will be present. These nonbeneficial changes can significantly contribute as a percentage to a person's overall illness or disease. In this patient, this included:

limited mobility of his shoulder,

limited mobility of his elbow to flex and extend,

weakness of his arm,

limited flexibility, movement, and strength of his third, fourth, and fifth finger, and

numbness of his face, particularly the corner of the mouth.

Once a nonstructural brain injury or nonbeneficial instinctual response is recognized, it can usually be treated successfully. Thus, the percentage that the nonbeneficial instinctual response contributed to a person's overall illness or disease can be eliminated. Many times this results in significant and noticeable clinical improvement.

You can clearly appreciate the difference between the traditional way of viewing stroke from a purely structural standpoint and the significant clinical improvement which is possible using this innovative pathway as a guide.

\* \* \*

### The Faulty Single Injury Explanation

The traditional way of viewing stroke is that there is essentially only a single structural injury. According to this view, an injury occurred due to a disruption or an occlusion of an artery supplying blood to a specific portion of the structural brain. The interruption of blood flow subsequently resulted in the tissue death or permanent dysfunction of the affected brain tissue.  This directly caused the development of the neurologic and neuromuscular deficits that people are frequently unable to overcome. This traditional way of viewing stroke centers on a physical or structural injury that occurred to a specific portion of the brain. Once all efforts to undo that structural injury have been attempted, you must live with whatever permanent dysfunction remains.

The major innovation of the neuroreactive pathway is that it greatly expands our understanding of stroke. This is because it disagrees with the traditional view that the neurologic and neuromuscular deficits are "solely" due to the disruption of blood flow leading to permanent structural brain tissue death and subsequent dysfunction.

**This pathway is a breakthrough in medical thinking because it shows the "permanent" brain dysfunction leading to the neurologic and neuromuscular deficits is not due to just one injury. It is due to <u>two injuries</u>.**

**The first injury involves the physical or structural brain. The second injury occurs in the nonstructural portion of the brain. More specifically, the second injury involves how the unaffected nonstructural brain responded in a nonbeneficial way to the actual physical structural brain injury.**

This is consistent with the following neuroreactive principle.

**The clinical symptoms that you suffer from stroke equal the sum of your**

**structural findings and injury**

**+**

**your brain's conscious reactions**

**+**

**your brain's subconscious beneficial instinctual reactions**

**+**

**your brain's subconscious nonbeneficial instinctual reactions**


**This concept of two simultaneous injuries, structural and nonstructural, occurring due to a stroke is not only innovative but revolutionary in medical thinking concerning this disease and other disease processes because its clinical implications are profound.**

At present, we are limited in our ability to clinically treat a stroke victim's structural brain tissue that underwent actual tissue death or was permanently altered, rendering it clinically nonfunctional. Symptoms due to actual structural brain injury will persist even if treatment is attempted. This same statement is not true of the nonstructural brain injuries that are experienced by stroke victims.

Fortunately, a large percentage stroke victims' ongoing neurological and neuromuscular dysfunction is due to the way the nonstructural brain responded to the actual stroke injury. This means two things are occurring. First, is that these individuals are under diagnosed because their clinicians have not recognized the possibility that a nonstructural injury is present. Second, they are under treated because no one has ever addressed the source of their ongoing dysfunction.

The typical stroke patient who meets this description is one who continues to suffer from limited movement and weakness despite years of therapy. These individuals want to make progress, but their nonstructural brain is preventing them from improving. The source of this dysfunction is the nonstructural brain injury and ongoing nonbeneficial instinctual reactions that are located in the subconscious mind. These nonstructural brain injuries can usually be overcome when treatment is directed at the specific area where the dysfunction is occurring.

**Using the above neuroreactive principles, a patient can expect to make a clinical recovery consistent with the percentage that the nonbeneficial instinctual reactions contribute to the ongoing symptoms.**

Effective treatment requires the ability to bypass the critical conscious thought process and correct the nonstructural injury. The goal of treatment is to eliminate the nonbeneficial instinctual responses in order to allow the subconscious brain to function the way it did prior to the stroke. The results are clinically impressive. People routinely regain their movement and function. The recognition and treatment of individuals in this manner may forever change the way we medically manage the ongoing neuromuscular symptoms caused by nonstructural stroke injury.

Sometimes the simplest treatments are the hardest to believe. This is because we are conditioned to believe that a successful medical treatment involves a "miracle pill" or a complex process involving some form of invasive experimental procedure. The simplicity of recognizing and reversing nonstructural stroke injury may not capture the imagination in the way that a very expensive new procedure would. The important thing is that the clinical results are life-changing for so many who have suffered ongoing neuromuscular dysfunction.

Another treatment benefit is the ability to clinically distinguish between ongoing neurological and neuromuscular dysfunctions due to the actual structural brain injury and those due to nonstructural brain injury. This will enable clinicians to more effectively target and address the remaining dysfunction due to actual structural injury.

**After Treatment:**

Jim underwent treatment. Immediately after, he discovered that:

1. He now has full mobility and range of motion of his shoulder. He is able to raise his arm and reach above his shoulder for the first time in twelve years.

2. The limited mobility of his elbow is improved. He is is now able to freely flex and extend his elbow.

3. There is increased flexibility, movement, and strength of his third, fourth, and fifth fingers.

4. The numbness of his face, particularly the corner of his mouth, is gone. Not only has normal sensation returned, but his face's muscle tone is improved as well.

Only the first two fingers on his hand did not significantly improve. This lack of improvement would indicate that further treatment would be needed to overcome this dysfunction. If there is no further improvement, the dysfunction in these two fingers would be attributable to an actual structural injury. Jim had achieved significant results in a single visit that are expected to only improve over time.

Once a patient has regained the use of a previously disabled extremity, it takes the brain only a short time to overcome the habit of relying excessively on the other functional extremity. Physical therapy or rehabilitative therapy will also be more successful after the ongoing nonstructural injury has been treated since the barriers limiting movement and dysfunction have now been eliminated.

### In Summary

The concepts and explanations presented should deeply challenge our beliefs concerning the brain's plasticity, or ability to change after a stroke. We need to look beyond the concept that cellular tissue death is the sole injury responsible for the neurologic and neuromuscular deficits that are experienced. When you consider that a subconscious injury occurs in conjunction with a structural injury, it becomes possible to go beyond relying on neighboring brain tissue to assume the function of the injured brain tissue. In my experience, it appears to be more clinically effective to retrain the subconscious thought process to overcome the dysfunction it experienced as a result of the stroke. This is based on the reasoning that once a stroke victim suffers a nonstructural injury, the result is a continuous nonbeneficial instinctual response characterized by immobility. Over time the brain attempts to recover from the acute structural injury, but the subconscious brain fails to recognize that movement is possible. Once the nonstructural injury is identified and addressed, movement once again is made possible.

# CHAPTER 8

*The Brain That Refused To Allow Itself To Recover From*
*Physical Injury*

Many people fail to appreciate that the brain frequently refuses to allow itself to recover from physical injury including trauma and surgery. The occurrence of these precipitating events can lead to the development of a distinct brain injury that presents as nonbeneficial instinctual responses, which directly contribute to the symptoms you may experience. This chapter allows you to understand that many seemingly untreatable physical injuries can now be overcome by addressing the hidden brain injury responsible for the ongoing dysfunction.

## The Importance Of Reason

Most people start their days by performing their daily routine. Their activities and interactions are usually predetermined and anticipated. Some individuals spend their entire day just going through the motions without putting much thought or effort into what they are actually doing. Perhaps you can recall a person who meets this description. One noticeable observation is that when these people are engaged in their routine day to day activities, they appear functional.

The word functional is another name for our brain's ability to stay in control. As long as the brain perceives that it is in command, it is much less likely to develop the symptoms that are associated with nonstructural brain injury. Our brains are continuously on guard for unpredictable events or challenges that may result in a potential loss of control. The inability of our brains to successfully respond to a potential challenge such as physical trauma can result in nonstructural injury. One tool that our brains use to prevent potential injury is making sense of things through "reason."

When the brain is forced to instantly react to a potential loss of control, it does not have the time to reason through correct decisions or proper responses to a given situation. This is what occurs when we are subjected to physical injury including trauma or surgery. When an instant response is needed, the subconscious brain, whose function it is to maintain control, provides the best one that it can give at that moment. Many times this instinctual reaction is not the thought out, well rehearsed, or optimal response that is required to prevent a total or partial loss of control.   The brain just responds with the goal of survival. The brain does not think about "what if" or "should I." All the brain can do is make a decision and live with its long-term results. Many times these split second decisions result in the brain mistakenly programming itself to respond in an instinctual nonbeneficial manner.

Neuroreactive medicine anticipates the development of this type of nonbeneficial instinctual response in the following principles:

**The greater the degree of injury or trauma, the more likely an individual will develop a nonstructural injury.**

**The shorter the time interval for the brain to respond to a physical injury or trauma, the greater the likelihood of developing a nonstructural injury.**

**Multiple traumatic events can cumulatively cause a nonstructural injury, while a single isolated event may not.**

*** 

In the following paragraphs, you will learn about the stories of several individuals. Their stories may even sound similar to your story or the story of someone you know. These people have something in common. They each underwent a trauma, physical injury, or surgery, yet their recovery did not go as they would have liked it to have gone. The reason is that they all suffer from a brain that refuses to allow itself to heal or get better.

## What Really Happened

The trauma these people experienced will challenge us to seriously rethink how we view the disability and dysfunction that result from a "purely" physical injury. What really happened is that these individuals' brains responded to a physical injury by suffering two separate injuries. The first occurred at the site of the actual physical injury. The second one occurred as a result of how the nonstructural brain adversely responded to the initial incident. When the second is present, it is seldom recognized because the patient's complication or disability is attributed to the physical injury. This is the same as mistakenly saying that the injury only occurs where it hurts. Those who are affected believe that their symptoms first became apparent after they experienced some type of accident, trauma, or surgery. Encountering such an individual whose injury did not improve after years of treatment should send up a red flag that a nonstructural injury may be present.

**Their nonstructural brain is continually responding incorrectly to an event in the past that no longer exists.**

These concepts are evidenced in the following cases:

## Phantom Pain, Post Traumatic Stress, Night Terrors, Amputation Site Pain

John, having recently started a new job, was working on a piece of industrial equipment for the first time. His arm was severely injured when it accidentally got caught in the machinery. He was taken to the hospital where it was determined that his arm was beyond repair and that an amputation needed to be performed. When John awoke from the surgery, he found that he had lost the portion of his right arm just beyond the elbow. Over the next three months, John attempted to recover. He received a prosthesis and underwent physical therapy, but overall, things were not going well. John continued to experience severe phantom pain. He felt constant excruciating pain emanating from the portion of the arm that had been amputated. It was as if his arm were continually being twisted, similar to the time when it was caught in the machinery. John was reminded of this experience each night when he tried to go to sleep. His night terrors and post-traumatic stress prevented him from moving on and fully recovering. John also felt significant pain on the stump of his arm where the amputation occurred. He also found it was difficult to wear or move his prosthesis. The pressure caused by the weight of the prosthesis made it very difficult for John to comfortably use it. For these conditions, John saw several caregivers, including his neurologist, his internist, his rehabilitative medicine specialist, and his psychiatrist. Despite correctly adjusting the prosthesis, the only thing further that could be done for him was to adjust his medications. Unfortunately, these measures did not result in any significant improvement or even a better night's sleep. The pain, suffering, insomnia, loss of functionality, night terrors, post traumatic stress, and phantom pain persisted.

These symptoms are not uncommon to many individuals who undergo an amputation as a result of a chronic illness or an accidental injury. The question that needs to be asked is, "How can you help these people overcome their symptoms when surgery, medication, physical therapy, and time are unable to provide improvement?" One-way to accomplish this is to recognize that a nonstructural injury is present in addition to the apparent physical injury. The presence of such an injury provides an explanation for patient's continual discomfort. The good thing is that nonstructural injury can be treated once it is identified.

John was referred to my office by a family member. When I met John, it had been three months since the time of his injury. He was wearing his prosthesis with difficulty and was taking four separate medications. These medications included a pain pill, a sleeping pill, and two other medications to enable his mind to deal with his present situation. John expressed that he had not made any improvement over the past two months. He said that he was told that there was nothing more that could be done but to give it more time and keep using the medications. When people experience phantom pain, night terrors, and post-traumatic stress, they are often unconsciously reacting to a past event that led to a loss of control. I was able to recognize from John's history that such a nonstructural injury was present and actively contributed to the symptoms he experienced.

Treatment was accomplished by eliminating the nonstructural injury that resulted from the loss of control he experienced from the accident and amputation. Afterwards, John said that I would not believe it, but his phantom pain was gone. He also noticed that there was no longer any stump pain; he could now comfortably move and operate his prosthesis. He did not even notice the weight and pressure from his prosthesis which had been a significant source of his earlier discomfort. I told him to come back in one week so I could find out how he felt. He returned one week later and was extremely happy with the improvements he had made. He reported that the night terrors were gone, and he was finally able to get a good night's sleep. He also mentioned that his phantom pain, post-traumatic stress, and his stump pain were completely gone. His wife was also very appreciative that her husband had made such significant improvement. I followed up with John approximately three years later. John reported that he was doing well and that all the symptoms that were treated never returned.

### Stabbing Pain, Pins And Needles Sensations, Surgical Site Hypersensitivity

Bill is an ironworker who started to experience abdominal pain under his right ribs. At first he ignored it, thinking it was probably something he ate. Eventually, he knew something was broken, so he had to get it fixed. His doctor immediately diagnosed him with a case of symptomatic gallstones or acute cholecystitis. He was sent to the hospital and underwent a laparoscopic removal of his gallbladder. The surgery was expected to require four tiny abdominal incisions. When he awoke, he found that he had a three inch scar in addition to the four little incisions. He was quite surprised and experienced severe pain. He was told that his operation was difficult due to scar tissue that required a larger incision to safely remove his leaking gallbladder. He remained in the hospital for three days before being discharged. When he followed up with his surgeon, he complained of constant painful sensations of pins and needles where the three inch incision was located. This area was very sensitive to deep pressure as well as light touch. Even the feeling of his shirt brushing against this area on his skin elicited extreme discomfort. His surgeon examined the incision and determined that it was healing quite nicely, so Bill was told to just give the area more time to heal. As the months went by, his symptoms did not go away despite the use of medications, injections, acupuncture, and a few other treatments. Bill was referred to my practice by a patient of mine. After hearing his symptoms and observing how painful his hypersensitivity was even to the mildest touch, I told Bill that it is possible to overcome these symptoms. I related to Bill that he appeared to be experiencing a nonstructural injury that occurred as a result of how his brain reacted to his surgery. This occurs when one physically recovers but his brain continues to adversely respond to a past event. I told Bill that it was unlikely he was experiencing nerve impingement or a hernia under the skin. I also mentioned that it was improbable that the nerves innervating his incision were disrupted or severed. It was important to relay this information since many affected individuals are frequently given mistaken information regarding the cause of their pain. Treatment was directed to the area that improperly responded to the surgery. The result was dramatic. The sensation of stabbing pins and needles immediately disappeared and did not return. The hypersensitivity was completely gone. Approximately one year later, Bill remained a very happy man who continued to be symptom free.

Hypersensitivity and the sensation of pins and needles occur quite frequently in many individuals. Once these symptoms are recognized as a nonstructural injury, they can be easily overcome.

**Chemotherapy Induced Neuropathy**

Jessica was told by her doctor that she needed surgery to remove an enlarged ovary. Ovarian cancer was discovered during her surgery and was removed, along with her uterus, fallopian tubes, lymph nodes, and other affected organs. She then received multiple courses of chemotherapy over the next several months. During this time, Jessica related that she developed discomfort in her leg. It was an occasional annoying burning feeling in her upper legs. The burning then progressed into constant sensations of burning pain and discomfort. She felt as if a hot coal was touching her lower legs and feet. She subsequently underwent an extensive diagnostic workup including, CT scans, MRIs, and neurologic evaluation. Since no structural causes were found to be present, her neuropathy was attributed to the aggressive chemotherapy she received. When the chemotherapy was discontinued, her symptoms persisted despite traditional medical treatment and rehabilitative therapy.

Jessica flew in from her home several states away to see if something could be done to improve the quality of her life. When I met her, I asked Jessica the usual questions.

Dr.: What are your symptoms?

Jessica: I experience a constant burning, stabbing pain in my lower legs and feet. It feels like my nerves are on fire as if I am being prodded by a hot coal.

Dr.: How long have you had these symptoms?

Jessica: They have been occurring for the last two years.

Dr.: What do you believe caused the symptoms?

Jessica: I am not sure. They have been present since I underwent chemotherapy for the treatment of ovarian cancer. They were not present after the surgery but developed while I was on the chemotherapy.

Dr.: What type of workup and treatment have been done so far?

Jessica: I have seen two neurologists as well as my oncologist. I've undergone extensive testing including CT scans and MRIs. The only thing I was told is that the neuropathy appears to be due to the chemotherapy. I've tried multiple different medications and have undergone several rehabilitative treatments. None of these have helped.

Dr.: So according to your many specialists, there is no specific structural or anatomic defect that is identified as causing your symptoms?

Jessica: "No."

It is apparent from these questions that Jessica's symptoms are not related to an ongoing structural issue from the previous surgery but rather to the chemotherapy. Her injury was due to the inability of her brain to overcome how the chemotherapy had adversely affected her. Her brain was continuing to react as if the chemotherapy was still present, even though it was not. This is consistent with a nonstructural injury. This diagnosis is sometimes not considered because this form of injury does not occur where the patient's symptoms are present. It also explains why her neuropathy could not be overcome using traditional medical or surgical interventions. These therapies do not treat nonstructural brain injury. Jessica's symptoms were eliminated in a matter of minutes when her nonstructural injury was addressed. They did not return over time.

### Persistent Numbness

Physical injury can cause a person's life to change in just the blink of an eye. Everything can appear to be going along just fine, and then a moment later you're suddenly injured. Many caregivers only focus their treatment on the actual structural area where the injury occurred. They fail to address the silent, nonstructural injury that involves the subconscious mind.

John experienced such an injury as a result of falling from a ladder. He knew that something was wrong as soon as he landed on his arm. His x-rays confirmed that his arm was severely fractured and needed to be fixed. His arm was immobilized in a cast and remained that way for several weeks. When the cast was finally removed, John noticed there was a large area of unexplained numbness around the site where his arm was injured. This numbness did not resolve despite treatment by his orthopedic surgeon or his neurologist. An MRI scan showed that his arm had healed appropriately without any structural deformity. When John explained his symptoms, I recognized them as nonstructural in origin. Numbness is frequently present when the brain continues to react to an injury that has previously healed.

John developed persistent numbness when his subconscious mind lost control and started reacting through ongoing nonbeneficial instinctual responses. Once these were eliminated, it was unnecessary for John to experience persistent numbness and the sensation in his arm returned.

### Fibromyalgia

Many people suffer from fibromyalgia. Fibromyalgia is a disease characterized by intense, constant, deep achy muscle pain. People who suffer also have painful joints and are unable to be comfortable in their own body. Nearly every touch or sensation of pressure produces achiness and pain. It is also quite common for these individuals to suffer from insomnia.

Cecelia experienced almost all of these symptoms for the last twenty years. She had given up hope that she could get better after being frustrated time and time again by treatments that failed to meaningfully help her. When I saw her for a routine exam and discovered that she had a diagnosis of fibromyalgia, I asked her...

Dr.: Who gave you this diagnosis?

Cecilia: My internist and rheumatologist.

Dr.: How many years have you suffered from this disease?

Cecelia: Twenty years.

Dr.: That's a very long time. What symptoms do you have?

Cecilia: I have constant deep achy muscle pain, painful pressure, insomnia, joint pain, and fatigue.

Dr.: When I squeeze your arm lightly in several places what do you feel?

Cecilia: I feel significant discomfort from pressure, achy muscles, and pain.

Dr.: As a result of my brief exam, I believe that you do indeed suffer from severe fibromyalgia.

Cecilia experienced a bicycle injury that occurred when she struck a large object and was thrown off her bike. Her symptoms appeared shortly after and progressed to the point where she constantly felt achy muscle pain, painful pressure, fatigue, insomnia, and generalized joint pain. Clinically, fibromyalgia appears to be a form of chronic nonstructural injury characterized by predictable nonbeneficial instinctual responses. An individual's symptoms will cease to exist when you remove these ongoing responses. This can usually be accomplished in a single visit. After treatment, all Cecelia's symptoms were completely resolved and did not return over time. Cecelia continues to be amazed that she can squeeze herself without any achy pain, pressure, nor discomfort.

## Rotator Cuff Dysfunction Despite Surgery

You never know how common a medical condition is unless you ask. When I started asking various individuals, I could not believe how many of them injured their rotator cuff to the point where surgical intervention was required. Surgery and subsequent rehabilitative treatment have helped a great many people improve their chronic pain, stiffness, and limited mobility. People who have undergone rotator cuff surgery usually say that they are 70% to 90% improved. In clinical practice, I rarely see someone who recovered 100%. Despite surgery and the best rehabilitation therapy possible, there are numerous individuals whose shoulders only have a certain range of limited mobility before reaching a point of stiffness. If the shoulder is moved any further in the same direction, that person will incur increasing resistance and significant pain. There is little that traditional medical treatment or physical therapy can do to get past this point of restricted mobility and pain. These individuals are left to learn to live with less mobility and just deal with the pain and discomfort. This is accomplished by restricting one's activities to prevent experiencing these symptoms. You may ask yourself if that is the way you want to live your life. I personally don't think so. The solution is to understand what is occurring to these individuals. Let's look at what is happening.

### How Rotator Cuff Injury And Treatment Contributes To The Production Of A Nonstructural Injury.

Prior to surgery, a person initially injures his or her rotator cuff musculature. This causes the person to suffer from pain with movement, limited mobility, and decreased functionality of the arm due to the structural injury. An additional injury also occurs when the brain adversely responds to the actual physical, structural injury. This produces an additional, nonstructural injury. In order to overcome the actual structural portion of the injury, people undergo surgery to the rotator cuff.

↓

Surgery helps remove the structural component of the rotator cuff injury. In addition, surgery can unintentionally produce a second potential nonstructural injury that contributes to the ongoing symptoms of pain, limited mobility, and decreased strength.

↓

This is because the act of surgery signals and challenges the nonstructural brain to respond to the surgical injury so that a temporary state of loss of control occurs in the subconscious mind. This is termed a

Nonstructural brain confusion

This reflects the brain's ability to respond to and overcome the loss of control due to the symptoms or dysfunction caused by the surgery.

Despite treatment, the subconscious, nonstructural brain is unable to completely resolve the loss of control. This leads to the formation of a

Nonstructural brain injury

A nonstructural brain injury then occurs due to the inability of the subconscious, nonstructural brain to resolve the loss of control, resulting in subsequent negative instinctual imprinting.

The outcome of this type of injury is that a nonbeneficial instinctual response is formed. From this point on, the portion of the subconscious mind that was injured will continually respond in an inappropriate way.

This type of injury may be clinically recognizable by the pain with movement, limited mobility, and decreased functionality that will be present. These nonbeneficial changes can significantly contribute as a percentage to a person's overall rotator cuff injury.

Once a nonstructural brain injury is recognized, it can usually be successfully treated. The percentage that the nonbeneficial instinctual

response contributes to a person's overall symptoms related to the rotator cuff can be eliminated. Many times this results in significant and noticeable clinical improvement.

From this pathway, we can understand why symptoms may persist even after corrective rotator cuff surgery. What is occurring is a brain that refuses to allow itself to get better due to an ongoing nonstructural issue.

The shoulder can be treated with further medication and various rehabilitative therapies essentially forever, and it will still not improve. That is why the above pathway makes a lot of sense. The pathway shows that therapy solely directed at the shoulder is treating the wrong area. Treatment that addresses the nonbeneficial instinctual responses produced by the nonstructural brain can correct the symptoms of pain, stiffness, and limited mobility. The results are life changing and are expected to be long lasting. This form of therapy can help individuals increase their mobility and eliminate pain from other joints as well. These would include the knee and hip joints.

### Lameness, Neuropathy, Neuralgia

I was seeing Rosie for a condition that would require pelvic surgery. When I performed an exam on Rosie, I noticed her husband was unable to move his arm at the shoulder. The arm just hung at the shoulder. Bob guarded his upper arm against touch and movement to avoid experiencing severe pain. I asked Bob what had happened. He replied that he had undergone a surgery involving a large, fatty tumor located in his armpit approximately three years earlier. During the surgery, it was discovered that his tumor had extended very deeply into his armpit. A more extensive surgery had to be performed in order to completely remove the tumor. Afterwards, Bob said that his pain that resulted in a very limited ability to move his arm at the shoulder joint. He also claimed that his armpit was so sensitive that he could not directly wash himself or place deodorant under his arm due to excruciating pain. Bob had followed up with his surgeon, several neurologists, and a neurosurgeon. He had even undergone extensive physical therapy to this area. After considerable diagnostic workup, including multiple imaging studies and consultations, it was determined that the injury was due to the extensive surgical dissection he experienced. The neurosurgeon felt that he had adhesions, scar tissue, or impingement of the nerves in the area where the surgery took place that would require a second surgery to correct. This surgery had considerable risks including the complications of continual pain, as well as additional loss of function. In the end, all that was provided to Bob were pain medications, but these did not seem to provide any relief.

Prior to the surgery, Bob had a job requiring physical labor. Since the surgery, he has been unable to work or make a living for himself or his family. His arm was essentially lame or nonfunctional. Bob suffered from loss of mobility, loss of use, loss of function, as well as from significant pain and suffering. His ongoing neuralgia and neuropathy was significant and unresponsive to traditional medical treatment.

I told him that his diagnosis was a nonstructural injury because his brain is continuing to react to the surgery that he underwent three years ago. I counseled him that I had seen his symptoms before and that they could be successfully treated. I told him to make an appointment with me.

One week later, he arrived in the office with his wife. I was able to address his nonstructural injury so that his pain and suffering were permanently gone. Bob was able to move his arm using a full range of motion in any direction. He had normal sensation to touch and all of his neuropathies were completely gone for good. I followed up with him one year later. He was still pain free and completely overjoyed that he felt normal once again.

There are many people who suffer, yet very little is done to help them overcome the devastation that they suffer. Once these symptoms are recognized as a nonbeneficial instinctual response, it is not very difficult to treat these patients so that they can lead normal lives once again.

## A Legal Argument

It could have been argued from a medically legal standpoint that Bob's symptoms were due to surgical negligence. That is the old way of thinking. Frequently, lameness, neuropathy, and neuralgia appear to result from a brain that refuses to allow itself to get better. Many cases that were previously attributed to surgical negligence are in fact due to the way the nonstructural brain adversely responded to an appropriate and uncomplicated surgical procedure. In the future, caregivers will emerge who are specialists in diagnosing and treating this form of injury. Their expertise should have a considerable impact on redefining what is medical malpractice as opposed to nonstructural brain injury.

## Amnesia, Traumatic Head Injury

Individuals can also suffer from a brain that refuses to allow itself to remember. This includes those who experience amnesia due to head injury. This type of injury commonly results from motor vehicle accidents. Some people experience a type of retrograde amnesia, or memory loss, of important events prior to this injury. I would like you meet one such person who experienced retrograde amnesia from this type of injury and was able to regain the ability to remember.

I was called to see Clarise in the emergency room for a medical issue. When I asked her a few questions, I noticed that she had difficulty recalling many events of her past. When I inquired why this was so, Clarise related that she was involved in a motor vehicle accident four years earlier. Since that time, she has experienced difficulty recalling memories of events that occurred prior to the accident. She has difficulty remembering math, the names of objects she sees, family, friends, and everything else. She finds it frustrating when she sees a movie for the first time with her family members, only to be told that she had seen the same movie twice before. She said that she has had to relearn everything since the accident. When she spoke, her face had a constant fixated stare, as if she was searching not only for the words but the proper order to put the words in prior to speaking them.

There are three possibilities that may be present.

The first is that the area of the structural brain that was actually injured healed a long time ago and a majority of the injury that is left is a nonstructural one. It is this injury that is preventing Clarise from accessing her memory. When memory loss occurs due to these circumstances, it is possible to achieve dramatic improvement.

A second possibility is that a significant ongoing structural brain injury exists in addition to a nonstructural injury. When this is the case, an individual may experience improvement when the nonstructural injury is addressed. The amount of improvement is proportional to the percentage that the nonbeneficial instinctual response was responsible for the individual's amnesia.

A third possibility occurs when an overwelming structural brain injury is present. In this situation, a portion of the brain that is structurally involved with the injury is so damaged that it cannot be used to regain a person's memory. When this occurs, the rest of the intact brain has the responsibility of making sure that it can still function in a manner that will allow an individual to be functional and physically survive. One way that this can be accomplished is for another area of the brain to take over the function of the structurally injured part of the brain. This may be physically possible based on the way the neurons of the brain are wired in close proximity to each other or are interconnected. The ability to accomplish this possibility is probably related to the extent, severity, and location of the structural brain injury. The more uninjured structural and nonstructural brain that is present to work with, the better off the patient is.

After the removal of the nonbeneficial instinctual responses that were present, Clarise had a calmer, more relaxed face when she spoke. It appeared that a great burden had been lifted from her mind. She was able to functionally recall her past. Her retrograde amnesia or memory loss had resolved. It was likely that the area of this patient's structural brain that was actually injured healed a long time ago and all of the injury that remained constituted the nonbeneficial instinctual responses that resulted in her ongoing amnesia. Clarise could not wait to show others that she could once again remember. She did so by asking a family member to question her concerning something that her memory loss would have prevented her from answering. Her family member asked her a series of questions that she would not be able to answer if she still had amnesia. She surprised this family member by being able to correctly recall the names, dates, events, and places of her past. She was deeply appreciative when she found that she had her memory back and could recall all the forgotten events of her past. Most importantly, she was functional once again.

# CHAPTER 9

*The Brain That Allowed Itself To Recover From A Surgery Before It Underwent The Procedure*

The previous chapter taught how it is possible to reverse nonstructural injuries. This chapter will discuss how to proactively prevent the formation of nonstructural injury. This innovative approach can allow the brain to recover from surgery before it actually undergoes the procedure.

## Arthroscopic Knee Surgery

Jim came into my office two days before he was scheduled to undergo an arthroscopic knee surgery to repair a large torn meniscus. He was counseled that three large punctures would be placed deep inside the knee to remove the tissue responsible for his pain and limited mobility. He was told that he would experience pain after the surgery. It could also take several weeks for him to feel better, possibly longer to regain full mobility. Jim was worried about experiencing the same pain, soreness, and limited mobility that many of his friends experienced after the procedure. Jim's goal was to avoid pain and recover even before he underwent the surgery.

## Is it possible to recover from surgery even before you undergo the procedure?

The answer may surprise you. The mind is capable of many great feats. One of these is to essentially recover from surgery even before the procedure occurs. You may ask how this could be. The answer is simply an extension of the neuroreactive ability not to feel pain when you are stuck with a needle. We have previously established that you only feel pain when the subconscious mind allows you to feel pain. It has also been discussed earlier that it is not very difficult to give an individual the ability not to feel pain to a needle stick even when the person is fully aware and awake.

Being able to recover from surgery before undergoing the procedure is simply an extension of the concept of blocking pain. The difference is that an individual undergoing the procedure can avoid reacting to the injury resulting from the surgery.

The subconscious mind perceives that surgical injury is similar to an accidental or physical trauma. The distinction between surgery and other forms of structural injury is that the individual is not consciously awake to experience the events that take place. It doesn't matter that a surgery was done to help you, to improve your health, or to remove the disease process that affects you. The mind interprets the surgery the same way in all three circumstances. Surgery is understood by the subconscious brain as an injury. When your body undergoes an operation, your brain will respond as if a traumatic injury occurred.

### Viewing Surgery As A Traumatic Injury

In order to understand this concept, just think about what happens when you undergo surgery. Your critical conscious mind undergoes a very deep level of relaxation through anesthesia. You are therefore unable to consciously respond to what happens during the actual procedure. During an operation, a structural injury occurs because we have to physically harm the body in order to enter it to remove or fix the internal structures requiring attention. By understanding that a surgery is essentially a traumatic injury, you can appreciate the events that unfold as a person is awakened from deep anesthesia.

When a person is brought out of anesthesia, the conscious mind is reawakened as well. It is then challenged to resume its job of responding to ensure that the body functions properly. As the conscious mind is awakened, it immediately receives pain signals from the nerves connected to the site of surgical injury. This area gives the conscious mind the report that a major injury has taken place. It asks the conscious mind to respond and do something to help overcome the traumatic injury. The difficulty of this challenge to react correctly can result in a loss of control.

The conscious mind experiences a loss of control when it is not prepared to react to the signals of traumatic injury it is receiving. When it is unable to handle a potential challenge, it sends the decision on how to properly respond to the subconscious mind. When the subconscious mind does not understand how to instinctually overcome the challenge, it can lose control. This results in the development of a nonstructural injury that will not benefit the individual's well being. The predictable clinical result after undergoing surgery is to experience severe pain. Prior to reversing the anesthesia, all the nerves are at rest and are unable to conduct responses to painful stimuli. This results in minimal to no signals of pain or painful stimuli during the actual surgery. When the anesthesia is reversed, all the nerves are free to tell the conscious and subconscious mind about what has occurred. The mind is then suddenly bombarded by a barrage of impulses signaling traumatic injury. This is similar to being hit by a baseball bat and having to deal with the sudden onslaught of pain. Many times, patients attempt to guard or protect the area of injury with their hands, but are unable to because they are strapped down to the table. Clinically it appears that patients are struggling. However, the patients are strapped to the table for purposes of safety. Being strapped down prevents patients from injuring themselves, injuring those around them, or, even worse, falling off the operating room table.

When the intubation tube is removed, patients frequently appear to be in a temporary state of shock, lying on the transfer cart moaning in pain and discomfort. These patients have experienced a loss of control, and their subconscious minds are working over time by instinctually responding in order to overcome the pain and discomfort. The consequences of the mind being unable to initially deal with the injury and subsequently losing control extends to recovery in the postoperative area as well as throughout the hospital stay.

Many people continue to experience significant pain, nausea, vomiting, chills, and uncontrolled shaking in the recovery area. When this occurs, they are routinely given more medication to counteract the symptoms that affect them. For example, if you have pain, you'll get pain medication through the IV tubing or intramuscularly through a shot. This is done so that your pain will briefly go away. You will become temporarily sedated so that you can sleep it off until it's time for the next pain shot to be given. This cycle continues until it is determined that you can do better with pills instead of IV pain meds or shots. Post surgical pain frequently results in your being confined in bed and unable to be in enough control to function for yourself. When you do get out of bed, the area where the surgical injury occurred hurts and limits your mobility.

Eventually, you are discharged from the hospital. It will still take some time for you to regain your sense of wellness and overcome the limitations resulting from the surgical injury you received. Many individuals continue to experience some of these limitations several years later. The clinical reality is that everyone responds to a surgical injury in a unique and personalized way. Many people go through an operation and do quite well. This is because their mind is able to regain control quickly or the symptoms of their injury resolve. Others are not so fortunate. They experience a difficult and sometimes prolonged recovery. Some never fully recover. Many people know of such individuals or have read about their experiences on the Internet. Frequently, these individuals attempt to discourage you from undergoing the surgery based on their own negative experience which they are still unable to overcome.

In summary, it appears that surgery is a traumatic injury that challenges the subconscious brain to stay in control. Failure to maintain control will set forth a predictable series of negative clinical events that persist until the subconscious mind regains control or the individual heals and recovers despite the efforts of the subconscious mind.

The inability to maintain control can produce a nonstructural injury from which the individual is unable to fully recover. As a result, the individual experiences ongoing symptoms.

Since Jim was going to undergo surgery in only two days, I treated him preoperatively using a neuroreactive approach and told him to follow up with me a few days after the surgery to see how he did. Jim came back to my office after the surgery. He related that his doctor told him that he had a very extensive tear in the meniscus that needed to be corrected. His physician had made three cuts in his knee in order to perform the procedure. After listening to what Jim said concerning the extensiveness of the procedure and observing the appearance of his knee, I concluded that Jim must have experienced a considerable amount pain and discomfort. I also believed that it would probably be very difficult for Jim to bend his knee fully or casually walk around. In fact, Jim claimed that the opposite was true. Jim said he did not have any pain after the procedure and did not even need to use any pain medications. Jim showed me that he could fully move his knee without any limitation and could also ambulate without experiencing any discomfort. Jim related that after the surgery, he felt as if the nerves innervating his knee were telling his mind that he should feel a lot of pain. In any other circumstance, he would agree with these neuronal signals and would have experienced severe pain. He then stated that the strangest thing happened when his mind started to be tempted to experience a sensation that he should somehow feel discomfort. He related that his brain instinctively responded that it was unnecessary to feel any pain or discomfort, so he did not. Jim thanked me for giving him the ability to recover from a painful surgery before he even underwent the procedure. He walked out of the office with a big smile on his face.

## Operative Laparoscopic Surgery

Natasha had a similar preoperative experience that allowed her brain to recover from surgery before she actually underwent the procedure. Natasha was going to undergo a laparoscopy to treat her chronic pelvic pain and endometriosis. Her pelvic pain had been present for several months despite the use of medications. It was anticipated that Natasha would probably receive two to three small incisions on her abdomen. I counseled her preoperatively that it is possible to overcome pain after surgery using an effective form of neuroreactive programming which would allow her subconscious mind to stay in control. I explained that when the subconscious mind remains in control, many people find it unnecessary to experience pain even after undergoing a major surgical procedure. Natasha was agreeable, so I talked to her and addressed the area of the subconscious mind that would be responsible for her post surgical recovery. It was then time for her to go into the surgery suite. Natasha underwent a procedure in which three incisions were made on her abdomen. The whole surgery took about thirty minutes. It included the dissection and removal of endometriosis. After I was done dictating the surgery, I noticed a peculiar thing out of the corner of my eye. I looked up and saw the familiar face of a person walking around. When I looked closer, I saw that it was my patient, Natasha. I was quite surprised, since most patients who have just undergone an operative laparoscopy are unable to get up immediately and stroll casually around. I walked over to her to inquire how she felt. She said that she felt perfectly fine and did not have any pain whatsoever. To verify this claim, I asked her again, and she said she had absolutely no pain. I checked to confirm that what she said was true by pushing very deeply into her abdomen where her pain was prior to the surgery, as well as in the areas where the surgical incisions were located. She smiled at me and said that there was absolutely no pain. When I followed up with her one week later, she continued to feel great and did not require any pain medications. It is amazing how your brain can allow you to recover prior to undergoing a procedure.

Barbara was scheduled to undergo a laparoscopic suspension of her vagina. It needed to be supported so it would not fall out. The surgery would be done laparoscopically using three incisions and would require extensive removal of scar tissue. Barbara had undergone neuroreactive treatment in my office for a completely unrelated issue in the past. I saw Barbara in the preoperative area. She seemed quite nervous and anxious about her recovery. She particularly focused on the postoperative pain that she would experience. I was able to address

Barbara's concerns using a similar approach that I used in the office. Barbara then underwent an advanced laparoscopic surgery to remove extensive adhesions and suspend the vagina. The procedure took an hour and a half. In the recovery area, Barbara was completely relaxed. She had absolutely no pain or discomfort even to deep palpation. One would expect that the portion of the body that just underwent a surgical injury which included extensive removal of scar tissue would probably hurt, but Barbara did not have any pain or discomfort. This amazing recovery was not lost on the residents and interns who were with me. They were amazed that Barbara did not feel any pain when they examined her and pushed on her abdomen.

Many people might claim that these patients were hand-picked, gifted, had special abilities, or were different from normal individuals. The words "normal individuals" usually translate to mean someone like yourself. The reality is that the individuals who are mentioned in this book are random, everyday normal people. They just want to feel better and avoid a painful recovery after surgery.

### A Surgical Correlation

Now let's consider the procedure known as a total abdominal hysterectomy. There are several minimally invasive techniques that can be used to perform a hysterectomy. For purposes of illustration, I'll discuss the total abdominal hysterectomy, which is the procedure that is consistently the most painful and difficult to recover from. This is a surgical procedure in which a five to nine inch incision is made on the abdomen in a horizontal or vertical fashion. After this is accomplished, the uterus and cervix are surgically removed and the abdomen, including the incision, is closed up. A hysterectomy appears to be rightfully understood as a major surgery that is a very painful procedure which usually requires a somewhat lengthy recovery. If you do not believe this statement, just ask one of your family members who underwent the procedure several years back and who is still recovering from the experience. People who have this type of experience know that once you're awakened from anesthesia, you experience a large range of sensations. These include nausea, vomiting, overwhelming pain, as well as the urge to breathe, even though a tube is still stuck in your mouth. When you are awakened from surgery, your body attempts to tell your subconscious mind that a major injury has occurred and that something needs to be done to overcome this injury.

In the recovery area, this scenario continues until enough medication can be administered and you are so medicated that you can be transferred to a bed to recover for a few days in the hospital. Since you have experienced an injury to your abdomen, you may find it difficult to be comfortable, move around, or control the other symptoms that may arise. These include nausea, vomiting, lack of bowel motility, lack of energy, and other symptoms. Some symptoms may persist for a long while, even after you've been discharged from the hospital. It is so disheartening to see an individual experience such suffering and discomfort. These individuals are forced to walk very slowly and appear slightly bent over. They also unconsciously use their hands to guard their incision. Perhaps I notice this because I view this type of painful recovery as unnecessary and potentially avoidable.

When total abdominal hysterectomy is performed on an individual who has been neuroreactively treated preoperatively, it is common to find that these people have significantly better pain control and speedier recovery. It is not unusual to be walking around the halls on the same afternoon of their surgery. These patients are routinely discharged the morning after surgery and can drive by themselves a day or two later. Several even return to work three or four days after undergoing a total abdominal hysterectomy.

The use of this preoperative treatment can enable individuals to recover in a much more comfortable fashion. This is especially true if the targeted therapy involves pain avoidance as well as promoting a faster recovery. The effects of preoperative treatment can be instantly seen as a patient wakes up from anesthesia. Individuals are calm and more relaxed. They do not struggle or have difficulty breathing by themselves in comparison to patients who are left to maintain control on their own. They do not experience the pain or discomfort exhibited by other individuals who do not receive this effective form of treatment.

In the postoperative recovery area, it is not difficult to observe how these patients are doing. You can easily identify patients who have undergone effective treatment because they're much calmer, more relaxed, and much more likely to be in control. When you see firsthand what preoperative treatment can accomplish, you can easily come to the conclusion that there is a better way that is available to everyone.

**An Explanation:**

It possible to provide an individual with the ability to recover from surgery before that person even undergoes the surgical procedure. This is explained using the following pathway.

**How The Brain Can Recover From Surgery Even Before A Person Undergoes The Surgical Procedure.**

Surgery

↓

Produces a structural injury causing physical symptoms

↓

↓ ← The additional negative effect of the reversal of anesthesia

↓

This signals and challenges the nonstructural brain to respond to overcome a potential loss of control due to the structural injury

↓

↓ ← The effect of neuroreactive treatment used prior to or
↓      during the procedure.

↓

Once the brain has been enabled to instinctually respond in a beneficial manner, it will do so whenever it is triggered. It is able to stay in control by not accepting the signals and challenges coming from the site of injury. The brain understood that these potential challenges leading to loss of control would be present at the time of surgery. When the brain has been enabled to respond instinctually, the brain does not have to succumb to the realistic risk of losing control.

↓

This leads to much speedier and more pleasant recovery as well as the continued normal functioning of the brain.

### Understanding Conscious Thought

In order to grasp the profound significance of this pathway, it is important to gain an understanding of how instinctually reacting and conscious thought relates to recovering from surgery. To understand this concept, you need to define what instinctual reacting means in terms of how the brain functions. **Instinctual reacting** refers to how the brain responds to something without even consciously thinking about what it is that it is responding to. The key words in this definition are "consciously thinking." When you instinctually react to something, you are bypassing the conscious thought process. Conscious thought interferes with your ability to instinctually react. You cannot instinctively react if you have to perform a detailed mental analysis to arrive at a decision. It is the conscious mind that is responsible for analytic thinking that prevents you from instinctually reacting in a beneficial way. You cannot instinctually react when your conscious mind is thinking in terms of yes or no, what if, maybe or maybe not, or should I or shouldn't I. All of these conscious thought processes lead to the same thing: delays in decision making, the total inability to make a decision, or a loss of control. These thought processes lead to the formation of a nonbeneficial instinctual response.

### The Beneficial Instinctual Reaction

It is the ability to instinctually respond to illness, physical trauma, or surgical injury by bypassing conscious thought that constitutes an innovative treatment frontier. This ability would allow caregivers to improve many conditions that could not be previously treated. Each day our subconscious brain is reprogrammed to instinctually respond to day-to-day events in order to maintain control and to function efficiently through the process of adapting and learning. Until now, many of us have had no need to even consider why it is we do so or what potential benefit these instinctual reactions provide us. One benefit is that instinctual reactions enable us to functionally respond to events that may challenge us without our losing control. The inability to instinctively respond in a correct manner may deeply hinder our ability to avoid or experience injury. There are countless examples that can be thought of. These include obvious ones as well as more subtle ones.

### The Rattlesnake Example

An obvious example of an instinctual response that clearly benefits us is the ability to recognize and instinctually respond when danger is present. Just imagine that you are walking in the woods and you suddenly hear a rattling sound getting louder, followed by a movement in the grass located a few feet in front of you. What do you do? You instinctually respond by reacting to the rattling sound and the visualized movement. You do not stop and consciously ponder the possibilities of what the sound and movement could be, as well as their intentional implications. You instinctively react, don't you? What is the benefit of doing so? The clear benefit is being able to avoid being injured and experiencing pain from the rattlesnake that is about to strike at you. What do you call the individuals who consciously have to think out a game plan of what to do prior to responding? You call these individuals "victims."

If you have difficulty overcoming rattlesnake poison and you cannot instinctually respond in a timely manner, you run the risk of a loss of control that may cause serious injury and possibly death. This is why individuals respond to this potential loss of control through instinctual reacting. It enables them to respond fast enough to successfully meet the challenge they are facing so that they can stay alive.

### The Handshake Example

A more subtle example of an instinctual response that clearly benefits us is the ability to be accepted and avoid being rejected by others around us. Frequently, this is done through the process of shaking hands. Just imagine what occurs when someone comes up to you and extends his or her hand outwardly to you. What do you do? Do you consciously think about what to do in this type of situation including examining the extended hand for creases in the palm to tell the person's fortune? Of course you do not. You immediately and instinctively grasp the person's hand with your own and shake it. How do we understand that responding in an instinctual manner will clearly benefit the individual who does so?

The answer to this is that a handshake is a nonverbal signal that is used to initiate communication as well as acceptance. A handshake is also a very complex way in which we communicate with touch. When someone extends a hand, the other person is obligated to grasp it and initiate the process of shaking hands. The opposite is true as well. Failure to instinctively recognize the ritual of handshaking will lead to the other person having feelings of rejection or confusion as to who the other person is. Remember the reaction to a common childhood prank when someone tried to shake your hand, but you moved away so that the other person's hand was left suspended in the air? You thought it was funny because the other person was just standing there with his hand suspended in the air, not knowing what to do. In reality, the other individual was experiencing a temporary loss of control due to the interruption of an instinctual reaction pattern that he was trying to complete. What you failed to realize after performing the prank was how the other person verbally and socially responded to you.

This response was one of rejection. This occurred due to the deeply ingrained belief that it is a warning signal when a person does not shake your extended hand. If a person does not immediately participate to reciprocate a handshake, then the person who fails to participate will be critically judged as someone who should be avoided and not trusted. A handshake is only a beginning or an invitation to initiate a conversation. Individuals who cannot perform a handshake correctly will be isolated or excluded from the more meaningful conversation that comes after the handshake. A handshake is like trying to get into a locked house with a key. Unless the key is used correctly, you will never get past the door and you will remain an outsider. Thus, a simple handshake is a subtle example of an instinctual response that clearly benefits us.

This is why beneficial instinctual responses are important. They protect us from danger and allow us to interact with other individuals. These same instinctual responses can be used to beneficially respond to a potential loss of control by being able to bypass conscious thought and instinctually react in a way that benefits our well being.

This is what occurs when an individual gains the ability to recover from surgery before even undergoing the actual surgery. When the anesthetic is reversed and the individual begins to regain conscious-ness, the brain is challenged to overcome a potential loss of control due to the traumatic surgical injury. The challenge to overcome the loss of control is quite difficult for the conscious mind to resolve. As a result, the decision of how to act and how to respond to the loss of control is left up to the ultimate authority for these decisions, the subcon-scious mind. When an individual's subconscious mind is enabled to correctly and instinctually respond neuroreactively through effective intervention prior to the surgical procedure, it can effectively deal with a challenge to it without losing control. It is the ability of the brain to instinctually respond that allows it to maintain control and over-come the neuronal signals that represent a potential loss of control. The brain is able to stay in control by overriding and not accepting the signals and challenges from the site of injury.

## Treatment During Surgery

This raises the question, is it possible to help an individual over-come surgical pain and avoid an adverse postoperative event even if we do not talk to the patient prior to his undergoing the surgery. In my clinical experience, the answer is yes. It is not necessary to provide preoperative neuroreactive input prior to the surgical procedure in order to help prevent a pain response or another type of adverse event from occurring. When you understand the pathway leading to a nonbeneficial instinctual reaction, you can see that surgery is a traumatic injury that can lead to a potential loss of control by the subconscious mind. If you look at what happens during surgery, you can easily determine that when patients undergo anesthesia, they are chemically relaxed so that their conscious minds will not resist by feeling any pain or discomfort.

When you realize this, you can understand that anesthesia provides a way to achieve direct access to the subconscious mind. This is accomplished by anesthetizing or chemically bypassing the conscious thought process. The subconscious mind never sleeps during surgery; it is always awake and ready to accept suggestions that will benefit it and allow it to maintain control. The same situation occurs to a lesser extent when a patient receives preoperative sedation.

In summary, when you receive narcotics or sedation, the doorway to the subconscious mind swings open and the opportunity exists to communicate directly with the subconscious mind. The difficulty medicine has is that many clinicians do not take advantage of this opportunity to impart the appropriate neuroreactive input to enable their patients to recover faster or feel better. Perhaps this is because most physicians are not even aware that this opportunity exists or don't know what to say when they find it does exist. I would like to show what can be accomplished when neuroreactive treatment is used while an individual is undergoing an actual surgery. The following is an example of the brain that gained the ability to recover during a surgical procedure.

### Vertigo

Pam is a patient who had to undergo an operative procedure that she had experienced a few times in the past. Every time she was awakened from her surgery, she experienced severe vertigo. Vertigo is a disease characterized by intense dizziness, as if the room is constantly spinning around causing an individual to be off-balance. Pam's vertigo usually lasts for about two weeks after each procedure. During this time she is unable to care for herself and is essentially forced to stay immobilized. She fears that if she moved, then she would experience disabling dizziness as if the room were spinning out of control. This vertigo was always present after surgery even if different medications or anesthetic protocols were used to prevent its occurrence. It was not unreasonable that Pam was hesitant about undergoing a surgical procedure that she needed. After I told her I would give her the preoperative neuroreactive input she would need to prevent the vertigo from occurring after the surgery, Pam finally agreed to undergo the procedure.

On the day of surgery, she reminded me to give her the suggestions that would allow her to remain in control so that she would not experience the impending vertigo. Just as I was going to talk to her, I received an urgent page to go to labor and delivery for an emergency C-section. I told Pam that I would talk to her during the actual surgery and give her the suggestions she would need to feel better and not experience vertigo. After the delivery of a healthy 10 lb. 3 oz. baby girl, I returned to the surgical area to find that Pam had just been taken into the operative room and was already prepped to undergo the surgery. After the procedure was over, I went over to the head of the bed and spoke to Pam who was still intubated with the tube hanging out of her mouth. You would think that a person who is still intubated cannot possibly respond to neuroreactive input, but individuals who are under an anesthetic do quite well since these patients' conscious thought process will not pose any resistance to the suggestions that are provided. After spending only a few minutes talking to her, I got paged back to labor and delivery for another emergent delivery.

When Pam followed up with me a week later, she had a big smile on her face and was very happy. I asked her why she was so happy. She said that her entire life she had experienced vertigo at least once a week. Since the surgery, she felt completely fine and had no recurrence of her vertigo. She was amazed that this was the only procedure that she was able to undergo in which the vertigo had not been there immediately when she was awakened. I told her that it would be very unlikely for the vertigo to ever return in the future. I followed up with her approximately two years later, and Pam was happy to mention to me that she continued to be free of any symptoms of vertigo.

This story is not unique. Caregivers have the opportunity during surgery to talk directly to their patients to help them feel better and recover faster after surgery. I've done this clinically over and over again so that my patients do not lose control or develop adverse clinical symptoms due to a nonbeneficial instinctual response. The results are consistent in that individuals undergoing surgery remain in control and do not experience the pain or the difficult recovery that patients who do not receive these suggestions experience.

**In Summary**

You can prevent the future formation of a long-term nonstructural brain injury by providing the preoperative input needed so that a loss of control will not occur. This is accomplished by providing the subconscious mind with the information and instructions that it needs so that the subconscious mind will know how to instinctively respond to the signals of injury resulting from surgery. When the subconscious mind is properly prepared and undergoes surgery, the subconscious mind will have the ability to overcome the urge to respond improperly due to a perceived loss of control. For example, many individuals who undergo surgery may be quite surprised to find that it is unnecessary to experience pain, discomfort, nausea, limited mobility, vomiting or other dysfunction after surgery. The result is that patients feel better and recover faster. Most importantly, it is unnecessary to experience the type of recovery that you hear about on one of those Internet sites in which people share their horror stories about undergoing and recovering from a procedure.

# CHAPTER 10

*The Brain That Avoided The Need For*
*Anesthesia During Surgery*

The concept of why suffer when you do not have to applies to procedures performed in the office as well. Individuals can undergo surgical office procedures comfortably without formal anesthetic. This can occur when the brain is enabled to react to a surgical procedure using beneficial instinctual responses.

The result is being so comfortable while you are undergoing a procedure that it is unnecessary to experience any pain. Since you do not experience any discomfort during the surgery, there is nothing to recover from after the procedure. Many people feel so good that they go out for lunch. Examples of these surgeries that I routinely perform include hysteroscopic tubal occlusion, which is a procedure that is performed to occlude the fallopian tubes to prevent future pregnancy. Another example of a surgery that is routinely performed in the office would be a hysteroscopic endometrial ablation. The purpose of this procedure is to burn away the lining of the womb in order to treat excessive bleeding.

This chapter explains how the brain can avoid the need for anesthesia during surgery. This is made possible by establishing beneficial instinctual responses in the subconscious brain prior to undergoing a procedure. Once this is accomplished, an individual's subconscious mind will be prepared to instinctually respond to challenges that could lead to a loss of control. It then becomes unnecessary for someone to experience any neuronal signals of pain or discomfort. This is appreciated using the following pathway.

**Enabling Individuals To Undergo Surgery Without The Need For An Anesthetic.**

Preoperative therapy establishes subconscious instinctual reactions to prevent being affected by neuronal signals of pain or discomfort.

Surgery (including office surgery)

Produces a traumatic injury or pain

This signals and challenges the nonstructural brain to respond to and overcome a potential loss of control due to the neuronal signals of injury or pain resulting from the surgery.

↓

The subconscious mind instinctually reacts, enabling the brain to stay in control. The brain does not accept the signals of pain or discomfort from the surgical site of injury. The brain has understood that these potential challenges leading to loss of control would be present at the time of surgery. The brain has successfully anticipated instinctually how to answer these potential challenges.

↓

This results in it being unnecessary to experience pain or discomfort. This leads to the ability to successfully undergo the procedure, a more pleasant recovery, and continued normal functioning of the brain.

You would think that it would be quite difficult to achieve such a deep level of control prior to undergoing such a procedure. It usually takes only a few minutes to accomplish this. The treatment is successful because both the physician and the patient are working together to achieve a successful surgery that goes smoothly. When you both work together, you can be successful nearly every time. Besides, it is rare to encounter an individual who is adamant about proving that he or she could not benefit by treatment to prevent the experience of pain or discomfort. What is such a person going to do, purposely feel pain to prove that he or she will feel discomfort? It just does not occur in clinical practice. To summarize this point, if you offered someone an easy pain free way or the harder more painful way, which one would you expect a person to choose? Clinically, most people who are about to undergo a procedure choose the easy, pain free way. After all, why would anyone want to experience pain when it is unnecessary to? This can be understood in the case of Mary.

Mary needed to undergo a hysteroscopic endometrial ablation. This surgery is indicated for patients who experience excessive uterine bleeding that is not due to a significant pathological cause. This procedure is performed by initially visualizing the inside of the womb. A disposable catheter is then placed into the womb and the endometrial lining is removed through radiofrequency ablation.

Mary was to undergo this procedure by my partner, but shortly before this procedure was scheduled to start, he was called away to perform an emergency cesarean section. Since Mary was already sitting in the waiting area, my partner stated that it would be okay if I performed the procedure. I said that I would have no objection to performing this procedure, so I walked into the room to meet Mary for the first time. Mary was a very pleasant individual who experienced excessive uterine bleeding throughout the month. A workup had been performed prior to this time and was completely normal. It is good practice for a physician to determine if there are any underlying risk factors that are present prior to having a patient undergo a procedure. This is especially true if the patient is one whom I've never met before. I asked Mary about her previous medical history. She related to me that she has had two cesarean sections in the past and has never undergone a vaginal delivery. She also mentioned that she had suffered from two strokes in the past, with her last one being less than five months prior to our contact. I asked Mary if my partner had mentioned how we would achieve sufficient anesthesia to perform the procedure. She said that all she was told was that I would be providing the anesthesia. My overall evaluation of this patient was that she had significant risk factors that included two cesarean sections and a history of recent stroke. The significance of the cesarean sections was that her cervix would be closed and would have to be dilated in order for me to be able to perform the procedure. Certainly a patient such as this would be a challenge for many gynecologic surgeons in the office setting. These surgeons would probably elect to perform the procedure in an outpatient surgical center or a hospital setting because of this patient's risk factors as well as the need for sufficient anesthesia to dilate the cervix.

I informed Mary that I would be happy to perform this procedure and instructed her that she would be receiving neuroreactive suggestion preoperatively which would allow her to be completely comfortable during the procedure. She was quite surprised when she heard my response. When she saw that I was serious, she did not offer any objection. I brought her back to the operative suite in our office and talked to her for approximately four minutes. When I was done treating her, Mary was able to achieve a deeply relaxed state and appeared to be completely comfortable. Mary then underwent the endometrial ablation procedure. I am presenting the steps listed in detail below so that you can appreciate what needs to be accomplished in the office setting. Perhaps you can imagine undergoing this procedure as described in the following steps:

1. A speculum is placed in the vagina.

2. The cervix is grasped with a sharp double pointed tenaculum (PAINFUL).

3. The cervix is dilated with dilators (VERY PAINFUL).

4. A hysteroscope is inserted inside the cervix and the womb (PAINFUL).

5. After the inside of the uterus is visualized, the hysteroscope is then removed.

6. The cervix is dilated further with dilators (VERY PAINFUL).

7. A large rod with a disposable mesh tipped catheter is placed and positioned inside the uterine cavity (VERY PAINFUL).

8. Once the rod is positioned, a radiofrequency current courses through the mesh tip which cauterizes and burns away the endometrial lining. This portion takes about ninety seconds. (VERY VERY PAINFUL).

9. The catheter is removed and the procedure is finished. Then the patient has to recover from the procedure and may experience discomfort, pain, and cramping (VERY PAINFUL).

As you would expect, Mary's cervix needed to be dilated in order for me to successfully perform the procedure. During the entire procedure, Mary was completely relaxed and comfortable. Her eyes remained closed, and there was absolutely no hint of pain or discomfort. After the procedure was finished, Mary was still completely relaxed and comfortable, essentially just sleeping with her eyes completely closed. When I awakened Mary from the procedure, she had no pain or discomfort and said that she felt perfectly fine in every way. When I specifically asked her if she had any cramping or pain, she responded that she absolutely did not. Since Mary felt perfectly fine, there was nothing to recover from. Mary was able to get dressed and walk out of the office having had quite a pleasant experience. Not only did Mary undergo a painful surgical procedure without any discomfort, she also avoided a significant number of commonly used preoperative medications. This included an injectable local anesthetic which is ordinarily used to numb the area around the cervix so that it can be manually dilated without significant discomfort.

Many practitioners who perform this procedure attempt to take away the pain by administering a combination of shots and multiple pain medications in a carefully selected patient.

This is a list of potential medications <u>that are avoided</u> when a neuroreactive approach is used.

**Medications to be taken one day before the procedure:**

1. **Motrin 800mg**: Take one pill orally every twelve hours until procedure (two pills).

2. **Cytotec**: Take one pill orally the night before the procedure in order to dilate and soften the cervix.

**Medications taken on the day of and during the procedure:**

1. **Motrin 800mg:**(a pain medication) Take one pill orally at break-fast on the day of the procedure (one pill).

2. **Vicodan Extra Strength:**(a pain medication) Take one orally two hours prior to procedure (one pill).

3. **Zofran 4mg:**(to prevent nausea) Take one pill orally one hour prior to procedure (one pill).

4. **Xanax .5 mg or Valium 5mg:**(to prevent anxiety) Take one pill orally one hour prior to procedure (one pill).

5. **Toradol 60mg:**(to prevent pain) Inject in deep muscle one hour prior to procedure, (one injection).

6. **Benadryl 50mg:**(to prevent anxiety and promote sedation) Inject in deep muscle one hour prior to procedure (one injection).

7. **B&O Rectal Suppository:** (Opium used as a pain medication) Place rectally one hour prior to procedure. Can use in place of Vicodan ES (one suppository).

8. **Hurricaine Spray:** (topical anesthetic) Spray on cervix to prevent pain.

9. **Lidocaine 1%:** (injectable anesthetic) Inject 20cc divided in four different places around the cervix five to eight minutes prior to the procedure (four separate injections).

10. **Additional Lidocaine 1%:** (injectable anesthetic) Inject additional anesthetic around the cervix if the patient has pain during the procedure.

**After the Procedure:** (Patient remains for twenty to sixty minutes)

1. **Toradol 30mg**: (to prevent pain) Inject in deep muscle after the procedure.

2. **Phenergan Suppository:**(for nausea) (another potential suppository)

**Medications to Take at Home:**

1. **Phenergan Suppository: (**for nausea)

2. **Vicodan Extra Strength:** (a pain medication) Take one pill orally every six hours after the procedure as needed for next forty-eight hours (eight pills).

3. **Motrin 800mg**: (a pain medication) Take one pill orally every six hours after the procedure as needed for next forty-eight hours (eight pills).

It doesn't take much to realize that there are a lot of potential medications that are needed for this procedure to be performed the "traditional way" so that the patient will be "comfortable." Futhermore, there is no guarantee that even if all the medications are given the patient will be comfortable during the procedure. A practitioner always runs the risk of a patient experiencing pain, anxiety, panic, fear, or a number of other unanticipated reactions to a procedure performed in the office. This is why <u>careful</u> patient selection is necessary for those practitioners who use the above regimen involving multiple medications. It is also noted in the commonly used protocols that it is very helpful to have a nurse hold the patient's hand and distract the patient with constant conversation during the procedure. The physician's role is to try to concentrate on performing the surgery as expediently as possible. After the procedure is finished, the patient still may experience significant pain, cramping, nausea, or other symptoms and may need to be monitored for up to one hour. It is also likely that further medication will be needed immediately after the procedure, which may be continued up to forty-eight additional hours.

**And the good thing is.... that this is considered PROGRESS because previously these procedures were only done in the hospital setting.**

Good things start to happen when we employ a preoperative neuroreactive approach.

1. Patients are more comfortable.

2. Numbness and anesthesia can be achieved through conversation that enables the patient to instinctually respond in a beneficial manner.

3. Patients are in a deeply relaxed "sleep" during the procedure.

4. Patients are so relaxed that there is no need for them to experience anxiety or panic attacks.

5. Patients are so comfortable that they do not require injections, shots, or many of the pain medications that were previously used to perform the procedure.

6. Patients will remain in a deeply relaxed state even after the procedure is finished so they have to be awakened to learn that the procedure is over.

7. Frequently, the patient will not remember undergoing the procedure.

8.  Recovery is instant and takes place as soon as the patient opens her eyes.

9.  There is rarely any post procedure pain or discomfort. Since the patient did not experience pain during the procedure, there is nothing painful to recover from.

1.0. The procedure becomes a pleasant experience for the physician and the office staff.

This is the result of a brain that gained the ability to avoid anesthesia during surgery. Patients are a lot more comfortable and require much less medication when neuroreactive suggestion is used. There is no need for preoperative medication one or two days prior to the procedure. There is minimal to no medication needed to perform the procedure.

It is also important to remember that these procedures can be performed without the need for a local anesthetic. You do not have to use lidocaine to numb up or anesthetize the cervix because patients are so comfortable that this step is unnecessary. There are very few practitioners who would even think of performing surgery without first injecting and numbing the patient with an anesthetic. I have not encountered nausea or vomiting either during or after the procedure so that medication for this complication is not necessary. Since patients recover instantly; there is no need to hang around the office for a lengthy period of time after the procedure. These individuals are so comfortable that they just get up, get dressed, and leave. When they are called later that day to see how they are doing, most report essentially no need for any type of pain medication. Many claim that they just go out to lunch following the procedure.

If a more invasive and complex procedure is required in the hospital setting, additional preparation will be needed in order to completely avoid anesthesia. This would include the combination of a more profound depth of neuroreactive suggestion as well as the ability of the patient to instinctually respond to any challenges leading to a potential loss of control. The reason for this is that there are many more variables, distractions, people interactions, as well as challenges that are anticipated in addition to the more invasive surgery itself. The key for a successful outcome is to simply prepare the patient prior to her undergoing the procedure. There are individuals who will do perfectly fine with just a single preoperative session, while others will need the benefit of additional preparation. It seems prudent to use several visits until the clinician is certain that the patient's subconscious mind has gained the ability to instinctually react to the anticipated surgery, in a successful manner.

# CHAPTER 11

*The Brain That Refused To Allow Itself To Overcome
Emotional Issues And Interactive Trauma*

Each day when I see patients in the office I am given the opportunity to understand a portion of their lives. Some people seem to go through life without experiencing any type of trauma, tragedy, or dysfunction. Their lives appear so perfect that casual observers might wish that they can switch places with these privileged people. Perhaps you have envied such a person at one time or another.

You may want to hesitate before you decide to switch places with that person. This is especially true when you remember that looks can be deceiving. Since we have learned not to look at the outside of a vessel but rather what is on the inside, it makes sense to at least give a glance or two at what is contained within the person. This is difficult for most of us because many people depend too heavily on their visual senses. They forget to use their ability to understand what they are seeing by listening or talking earnestly to whomever their eyes envy the most. Perhaps they need to rely more on x-ray vision. Fortunately, many caregivers do not have to use x-ray vision because patients readily let us know what lies inside if we ask them. It is this glimpse might potentially scare away those who look only at appearances. That's why the issues that negatively affect an individual are hidden. Sometimes these issues are so well hidden that the individual who has them forgets the issues are there as well as their underlying cause. Maybe these individuals do this so that they will not scare themselves away. Perhaps, it is too uncomfortable to relate to these issues while having to truthfully deal with one's self. Addressing these issues can cause much pain and suffering because they are tied to an interaction or emotional injury that was previously experienced.

These issues are so well hidden that a casual observer may notice that whenever a certain set of events or a specific situation arises, the subject instinctively reacts to it.  These reactions take the form of the likes and dislikes that help shape an individual's personality. Occasionally, a person's predictable instinctual reactions to a set of events or given situation appear to be a little peculiar.  In extreme cases, it is apparent to others that this person is not acting "normal." The individual is not reacting the way those watching would think or react.  It is as if the person is stuck in time and is reacting to an event that has not been present for quite some time. Some people view this as responding to a type of post traumatic stress.

A more innovative way to understand what is occurring is to consider that this individual has experienced an interactive, nonstructural injury characterized by a loss of control that led to the formation of a nonbeneficial instinctual behavioral response. Once a nonstructural injury is present, a person will predictably and instinctively respond in an abnormal fashion whenever a precipitating event or stimulus arises.

It is easier for most individuals to provide an excuse for these abnormal thoughts or behaviors than it is to address the underlying dysfunction.  One needs only to provide a medical name to an abnormal behavior in order to legitimize it. This label results in an individual becoming acceptable to others, even if that individual's thinking or behavior appears a bit odd.

A common example is if you react as if you are frightened of something and 99.9% of everyone else is not. This means that 99.9% of the people would think that it is peculiar for you to be reacting so differently from everyone else.  Now if you're able to give this unusual reaction a medical name, you can legitimize or justify your unusual reaction or behavior.  When you accomplish this, it's not you who is frightened or scared of something when everyone else is not. You become a medical condition called a "phobia." You are now expected to react abnormally because "you just can't help it." You can further justify your medical disorder by giving it a really complex name that is probably difficult to spell, pronounce, or even understand without the aid of a medical dictionary.

**A Handy Example**

An example of this occurs when someone comes up to you, shakes your hand, and then looks down at his own hand and says, "I better go wash it right away." You would probably wonder what was so toxic about a simple handshake that this person needed to wash his hands immediately.  You may even look at your hand to make sure that it looks clean. When you glance back up, you may even see the other person has just returned from washing his hands.  Now imagine your thoughts and reaction when this other individual tells you not to worry; it was only a little automyophobia (fear of getting dirty). Once you understand what the medical name implies, you can understand the odd behavior.  The funny thing is that you accept this person's unusual behavior because it is an actual medical condition that is perceived as something that cannot be helped or consciously overcome.

These medical names, symptoms, or behaviors have one common theme. They are forms of interactive injuries. This form of injury occurs when we are negatively affected by a potential loss of control that is not the result of actual disease, illness, physical trauma, or surgery. Interactive injuries are due to actual or perceived events.  This type of injury occurs because of an individual's inability to cope, adapt, or effectively respond to the interactions or stress that we are exposed to.  When we are unable to meet day-to-day challenges, we run the risk of losing control. This can lead to the development of a nonstructural injury.

**The Relationship Between Our Interactions, Emotions, And Actual Physical Trauma Or Disease**

Many people mistakenly think that interactive or emotional injury is completely unrelated to injuries that occur as a result of a physical trauma or disease. All of these injuries are intimately related because of the way the nonstructural brain responds to the potential loss of control. This is consistent with the following neuroreactive principles that show how the brain clinically functions.

**The nonstructural brain responds to loss of control predictably, regardless of its source.**

**It does not matter if the loss of control is from an illness, physical trauma, or an interactive injury; the nonstructural brain uses the same pathway to respond to each of these.**

This is not how a traditional medical approach views these conditions. The traditional medical view separates these injuries by subspecialty. If there is a structural or physical deformity, it will be in the realm of surgery to fix it. If the problem is due to a disease or illness, it will be dealt with by internal medicine or family medicine. Finally, if it isn't an illness, disease, or something that can be fixed with surgery, it is obviously one of those…you know… psychiatric issues. Many times, these "issues" are mistakenly dismissed as those which cannot be helped by the everyday caregiver. These issues can be addressed as being due to a brain that refuses to allow itself to overcome the emotional issues and interactive injuries that it has experienced in the past.

**This form of emotional and interactive injury is clinically expressed as ongoing instinctual nonbeneficial responses.**

Fortunately, the nonstructural brain does not deal with or even care about medical specialties or medical politics. All the nonstructural brain knows is that it has to meet the challenge to overcome a potential loss of control whenever one arises so that it can effectively ensure that the body functions properly.

Since we have formulated the innovative idea that the nonstructural brain responds to interactive injury using the same pathways as it does for disease, illness, or structural injury, it is time to explore what makes up an interactive injury.

## Understanding Interactive Injury

An interactive injury is one that results from our experiences, including those that are real or perceived due to our surroundings, other individuals, or even ourselves. Interactive injuries are due to the way we are affected by everything that we come in contact with. Sometimes we are even affected by things or events that we were never actually exposed to. The list of interactions that can have a potentially negative effect on us is endless. These injuries are frequently due to the needless cruelty of other people, especially those who are supposed to love us the most. They may also be due to friends, even though a good friend is defined as an individual who would not hurt another good friend. The following is a list of some of the infinite number of reasons that interactive injuries may occur:

| | | | |
|---|---|---|---|
| stress | embarrassment | taunting | teasing |
| name calling | fear | physical abuse | malicious lies |
| emotional abuse | rejection | not being included | verbal abuse |
| appearance issues | peer pressure | abandonment | neglect |
| guilt | blame | being unloved | performance issues |
| isolation | handicaps | hurt | physical deformities |
| molestation | inappropriateness | deprivation | broken trust issues |
| cruelty | being different | "good" parenting | family issues |

| | | | |
|---|---|---|---|
| self esteem issues | perceptions | popularity issues | different beliefs |
| distorted values | disappointment | traumatic stress | learning disabilities |
| coping difficulties | hate | mental trauma | inferiority |

Even though our interactive experiences can be bad, there is always the opportunity to overcome them. It is not necessary for these experiences to affect us negatively. This is shown in the following pathway.

### How The Nonstructural Brain Effectively Responds To A Potential Interactive Injury

The state of being good enough and in control

↓

And then being subjected to a potential interactive injury (listed above)

↓

This signals the nonstructural brain to respond to the potential emotional or interactive challenge so that a state of loss of control occurs. This is termed

↓

Nonstructural brain confusion

This is the brain's ability to respond to and overcome the loss of control by understanding what went wrong, being able to adapt, learning from mistakes, correcting any mistakes, doing better next time, and remaining good enough.

↓

The brain is able to respond by learning and adapting to regain control.

↓

This leads to recovery and normal functioning of the brain.

This allows an individual to stay in control, and more importantly, continue to be good enough.

This pathway shows that we can allow our interactions to negatively affect our wellbeing as well as prevent them from doing so. We prevent the negative effect by coping, adapting, adjusting, and learning how to change.

## Being Good Enough

Janie is a nineteen year old who saw me in my office concerning a routine issue. When I asked her about her history, it emerged that she had a very deeply troubled childhood. Her parents had abandoned her when she was very young. She then found herself being passed off to different relatives and caregivers. These foster parents never showed her much affection, nor did they include her in their family activities. Many times she was verbally and physically abused. She was told that she was not good enough and that she would never amount to anything. These "caring" individuals routinely pointed out her personal shortcomings in an attempt to embarrass and humiliate her. She was beaten and sometimes even burned. She was also told on a daily basis that her only useful purpose was to clean things and work as a type of indentured servant. This humiliation lasted for a number of years until she was grown up and able to go out on her own. When I talked to her, she appeared completely unaffected by her past ordeals. Her voice sounded perfectly fine in every way. She even said that she was entering college and was studying to be a psychologist in order to help emotionally troubled children.

Over the years I've seen thousands of people, yet this individual stood out from the rest. Janie had the most miserable childhood and was clearly abused. She had been beaten down both emotionally and physically, yet she appeared cheerful and extremely happy. She did not have any of the emotional scars, dysfunctional personality traits, or behavioral changes that I would expect from someone who experienced what she had been exposed to. It was as if I were talking to one of those hidden saints that we read about. Since this person appeared to be too well adjusted, I asked her the following question. "How can you still be perfectly fine despite everything you went through?" She looked at me and thought for a moment. Then, with a smile on her face, she gave the most amazing answer. She replied that all the abuse that she had experienced had actually no lasting effect on her. She said, "I did not believe what they said about me because on the inside I knew that I was good enough and I did not let anybody convince me that I was not." I was deeply impressed by the profundity of this answer and the inner strength that this person possessed. I wondered how many other individuals could endure what she had gone through without being negatively affected or suffering deep emotional dysfunction.

This leads us to think about what being good enough is. One way to look at being good enough is having the ability to not let ourselves or other people get in the way of our being ourselves. Being good enough can also be influenced by our interactions, experiences, or perceptions, including those that can prevent us from remaining true to who we are or those that can change the way we instinctively respond to ourselves or outside stimuli. For some, being good enough is a constant battle of maintaining control and not being negatively affected by potential emotional or interactive injuries. Others instinctively know that they are good enough and are completely unaffected by potential interactive injury even in the face of the seemingly insurmountable horrors that life may throw at them. Janie, in our example above, is one such person. Despite undergoing significant abuse and daily torture, she remained good enough to not give in and become negatively affected by her past experiences. She understood that not only was she good enough, but that things would eventually get better. This way of thinking and reacting to interactive injury is reflected by the simple but powerful words of the eighteenth century sage, Nachman of Bratslav. He taught…

1. Never give up….

2. If tomorrow is not going to be better than today, then what need do you have of tomorrow.

3. Life is like walking on a very narrow bridge: the key is not to be afraid.

4. It is a great thing to always strive to experience joy and happiness.

5. And finally...If you believe that things can be bad, then you have to believe that things can also get better.

Since it is not possible for everyone to meet the challenge of a potential interactive injury, some individuals will be deeply affected. In clinical practice, however, it seems as if everyone (except oneself, of course) is affected in some fashion by an interactive injury. Some people are less obviously affected, and others are more obviously affected. You do not have to be a rocket scientist to tell one from the other. The more you get to know a person, the more you are able to discover the effect that an emotional or interactive injury had on the way that person behaves and functions. The following pathway shows how the nonstructural brain is negatively affected when it is unable to respond to and cannot overcome a potential interactive injury.

**What Occurs When The Nonstructural Brain Responds Incorrectly To A Potential Interactive Injury**

State of being good enough and in control

↓

The effect of experiencing a potential interactive injury

↓

This challenges the brain to respond, creating a temporary loss of control. This state is termed

↓

Nonstructural brain confusion

This is the brain's ability to respond to and overcome the loss of control by understanding what went wrong, being able to adapt, learning from mistakes, correcting any mistakes, doing better next time, and remaining good enough.

↓

Despite its best attempt, the nonstructural brain is unable to completely resolve the loss of control. This leads to

Instinctual imprinting

This results in some portions of the subconscious, nonstructural brain remaining in control and remaining unaltered and unaffected by the emotional or interactive injury.

Other portions of the subconscious, nonstructural brain are now overridden or reprogrammed by the process of instinctual imprinting. This leads to the formation of a…

Nonstructural brain injury

A nonstructural brain injury occurs due to the inability of the subconscious, nonstructural brain to resolve the loss of control and the subsequent negative instinctual imprinting that occurs.

The result of this type of injury is that a nonbeneficial instinctual response is formed. From this point on, the portion of the subconscious mind that was injured will instinctually respond in an inappropriate way.

↓

This type of injury may be clinically recognizable by the abnormal or undesirable behavioral changes that will be present.

↓

Once nonstructural brain injury is recognized, it can usually be successfully treated.

**What does this mean to me?**

We fail to realize that we are continually reacting to our past when nonbeneficial instinctual behavioral responses occur. When we are stuck reacting to our past, we cannot achieve our full potential in the present or the future until we address the nonstructural brain injuries that exist. The issue of why so many individuals initially lose weight after dieting or undergoing gastric bypass surgery and yet regain it over time is a relevant example of this type of nonbeneficial instinctual behavioral response. This topic will be thoroughly covered in a subsequent chapter.

Individuals who experience nonstructural brain injury do not learn from their past mistakes, so they repeat the same mistakes whenever these responses are triggered. They are stuck responding repeatedly in the same abnormal way. These people become unable to consciously change because they are reacting instinctively. If you're not consciously aware of how you're reacting, you cannot see that you are responding and behaving differently than everyone else. Many individuals just live with the limitations resulting from nonstructural brain injury. These people just put up with their limitations, especially if these are barely noticeable. These individuals can worsen over time. They may develop significant physical symptoms or interactive dysfunctions that are clearly obvious to themselves and everyone else around them. When this occurs, there is general agreement that something is broken and needs to be fixed. The problem is that the affected person can not consciously fix what is broken. Frequently, too much time has elapsed since the abnormal symptoms or behavior first started. The affected individual has long forgotten what it was that he or she was abnormally reacting to. An affected person who suffers would consciously change if they could do so. No one wants to suffer abnormally when it is unnecessary.

The pathway that leads to the formation of a nonbeneficial instinctual behavioral response shows not only how these injuries develop but also that these injuries reside in the subconscious mind of the nonstructural brain. When the subconscious mind is unable to overcome the potential interactive loss of control, the affected individual continues to suffer until the injury is addressed. The good thing is that these injuries can be treated once they are recognized. This has been shown in clinical practice. The following are just a few examples of individuals who were able to regain the ability to deeply improve their lives.

### Tics (Uncontrollable Neuromuscular Behavior)

Raymond and his wife came to my office for discussion concerning a surgery that his wife needed to undergo. His wife's upcoming surgery was addressed in a positive, reassuring tone since the minimally invasive surgical procedure I proposed would allow his wife to overcome her illness. During our visit, I could not help but notice a strange tic that Raymond was unconsciously displaying. His right leg and foot were not just shaking back and forth; they were literally tap dancing while his left leg remained perfectly still. This scene was quite apparent to all in the room. It is very common to casually move or shake your leg or foot. People who commonly shake a leg and foot do this in a self-limiting fashion and have the ability to start and stop the process because they are in control. People effectively maintain such control in social situations so that they do not call unwanted attention to themselves. A tic may develop when a person loses control of the ability to start and stop a series of neuromuscular movements. In this case, it was the uncontrollable noticeable dancing movements of the leg and foot. Just imagine that you're watching one leg just dancing away while the other leg is sitting perfectly still wondering why it's walking partner is dancing when there is no music playing. Since I was curious, I asked this gentleman the following:

Dr.: How long has your leg been acting like this?

Raymond: It has been moving around uncontrollably for about six months.

Dr.: What happened six months ago?

Raymond: I was let go from the job that I had for the last fifteen years, without warning.

Dr.: Does it bother you that one leg dances around uncontrollably?

Raymond: I just live with it, but it does get in the way of interacting with people and interviewing for work.

I told this gentleman that his condition was quite common and I've seen and helped quite a few individuals overcome this type of dysfunction. Now let's summarize what was occurring. This individual was displaying an uncontrollable neuromuscular behavior or tic. This behavior had not gone away since it began six months earlier. Prior to that time, Raymond was perfectly fine and did not have any dysfunction. The only difficulty he experienced was that he was suddenly fired from his long-standing job. This individual's diagnosis is a tic due to a nonstructural brain injury. Apparently, the sudden loss of his job allowed him to experience a loss of control that resulted in a tic. This tic will not resolve and will be ongoing until the cause is addressed. Once we recognize that a person's symptoms are due to such an injury, it is usually not very difficult to successfully treat this type of condition. This patient underwent neuroreactive medical treatment that reversed the nonbeneficial instinctual behavioral responses located in his subconscious mind. The whole treatment took approximately eight minutes. After treatment, his tic was gone and would not return, even when the subject of his former job was brought up. One year later Raymond was still completely asymptomatic.

## Panic Attacks, Anxiety, and Seizures

Juan had suffered for years from anxiety, seizures, and panic attacks. The anxiety and panic attacks were characterized by an overwhelming fear that he was going to die. This produced feelings of weakness and fatigue. They frequently occurred when Juan traveled to new places. Juan did not have any idea why these conditions were occurring. At age fourteen, Juan first experienced seizures characterized by uncontrollable thrashing movements. A neurologist worked up these seizures, and no specific reason was given for their occurrence. Various medications were prescribed to treat Juan's condition.

When a neuroreactive approach was employed, Juan was able to clearly visualize and recall the events from his past that had bearing on his present. This memory was associated with a loss of control that he experienced as a child. He remembered that when he was eight years old, he felt terrorized by his alcoholic dad's uncontrolled temper and abuse. His drunken father frequently told him that he hated him, so Juan was forced to seek safety by hiding in his back yard tree fort. The tree fort was an ideal place since his father was too drunk to notice him. Since his father drank too much, he was unable to physically climb up to the fort to hurt Juan. The abuse continued until Juan was fourteen years old. At that time his drunken father was involved in a fatal motorcycle accident. Juan somehow felt personally responsible for his father's injury. Juan's perceived inability to reach his drunken father in time to save him from the accident led to another loss of control, causing seizures that progressed into panic attacks. During treatment, Juan became aware that his brain was still reacting to a series of events that happened many years earlier. His subconscious brain now realized that the anxiety, panic attacks, and seizures were actually nonbeneficial instinctual behavioral responses. His subconscious mind understood that his father's abuse and the motor vehicle accident were not events that he could possibly have changed; consequently, he was not responsible for their occurrence. Once these nonbeneficial instinctual behavioral responses were eliminated, Juan found it unnecessary to experience any form of anxiety, panic attacks, or seizures. Two years later, Juan remained able to go to new places and do new things without being bound by the negative effects of his past.

### Self Blame, Grief, Guilt, Binge Eating, And The Inability To Forgive One's Self

Brandy found out she was pregnant at a time in her life when she least wanted to be pregnant. She had just started school to obtain a degree so she and her two kids would be financially able to move out of her grandmother's house. The last thing that she needed was an unplanned, unwanted pregnancy. The unexpected news that this was a twin pregnancy only made things worse. When she told her boyfriend about the pregnancy, he was in denial and moved out of her life. Being a single mother with limited financial resources, the prospect of having to take care of twin newborns had a negative effect on Brandy's emotional state. She became increasingly depressed and expressed doubt concerning her ability to meet the challenges ahead. She began to verbalize these doubts, making statements like, "I wish that I never got pregnant" and "I did not want this pregnancy in the first place." It was a way of verbally and emotionally rejecting the pregnancy.

Many people commonly behave this way, but in this instance Brandy had an unexpected occurrence. Her ultrasound at twenty weeks showed that both her babies' heartbeats had stopped due to an umbilical cord entanglement accident. The news hit Brandy like a ton of bricks. The two lives that she had been carrying and that had been previously moving inside her were no more. They had been suddenly taken away from her. She was deeply saddened over the loss and felt very upset that she had said such negative things about her unborn children with whom she had already unconsciously bonded. She blamed herself for her babies' demise. After undergoing the delivery of her twins and going through the grieving process, she claimed she was okay. She would try at a later date to get pregnant once more.

One year later, I saw her in the office. She explained that for eight months she had been attempting to get pregnant but could not conceive. One look at her showed that things were not well. Brandy had still not been able to forgive herself for the loss of her twins. She felt that she deserved to be punished for the negative feelings she had about them at the time the twins died. Because of this, she was still instinctively reacting to a part of her past that was negatively affecting her present. She had developed a nonbeneficial instinctual behavioral response that resulted from a loss of emotional control. This loss of control resulted in a portion of the nonstructural brain becoming negatively imprinted in attempting to deal with the ongoing self-blame, grief, and inability to consciously forgive herself. Once her nonstructural brain injury developed, she was continuously reacting in an abnormal manner that had a profoundly negative effect on her daily existence. She continued to experience feelings of fatigue, guilt, regret, as well as exhibiting sudden outbursts of tears whenever she remembered her twins. She also felt the constant urge to eat, so she experienced significant weight gain. I understood why she was gaining weight, so I asked her the question, "Are you gaining weight because you need to suppress your feelings of loss and grief?" She thought about it and was able to relate her binge eating with her sad memories. I told her that a neuroreactive approach would allow her to eliminate her ongoing emotional pain and suffering. The memories of her past events would always be there, but these memories would have absolutely no effect on her. They would merely be memories. As the tears continued to roll off her eyes, she said she would like to finally overcome what had been troubling her for so long.

Brandy underwent a single session that addressed the nonbeneficial instinctual behavioral responses responsible for her symptoms. Afterward, she was able to feel the way that she should. She was able to recall the loss of her twins without experiencing the guilt, sadness, or self blame. She also found it unnecessary to eat inappropriately, since the underlying impulse was no longer present. She was finally able to move on with her life in a positive way. Two months later, she came back to the office and was happy to announce that she was pregnant.

### Other Fixations, Fears, and Hypochondriasis

Juanita was a fifty year old female who was undergoing testing of her urinary system. She needed to undergo a cystoscopy, a procedure that allows visualization of the inside of the bladder though a small scope. It's a simple office procedure that only takes a few minutes to accomplish. When Juanita heard that she needed to undergo this procedure, she had an interesting question or two that she felt compelled to ask me.

Juanita asked, "Why do you want to look inside the bladder?" "Do you think that cancer is present?" "Do you believe that there's something abnormal, but you are just not telling me?" Juanita didn't even wait for an answer because she started to react to the fear and suspicion that had previously negatively imprinted her subconscious mind. She continued asking question after question. "I know it is cancer." "You know there is cancer, don't you doctor?" "You don't want to tell me yet?" "I know I have cancer." "Cancer...Cancer... Cancer..."

At this point, it was obvious that Juanita had a nonstructural brain injury and was displaying a nonbeneficial instinctual behavioral response. Her nonstructural brain injury was an uncontrollable fixation and fear of cancer, which is essentially a form of hypochondria. After about twenty more cancer statements verbalized in under thirty seconds, it became quite apparent that she needed some help to overcome her dysfunction. Since she was unable to regain control, I decided to help her out a little. I told her that it was time to regain control and immediately proceeded to treat her underlying neuroreactive injury.

The first step involved bypassing the conscious thought process. This allowed Juanita to regain enough self restraint so that she stopped verbalizing about cancer. The next step involved addressing and correcting the nonbeneficial instinctual reactions responsible for her fears, fixations, and hypochondriac outbursts. After treatment, she was consciously back in control. During the treatment, she was able to recall the real reason why she reacted uncontrollably to the suggestion or thought of cancer. She related that ever since her mother developed a severe form of metastatic breast cancer, she could not handle the thought of reliving her mother's experience. Her mom's cancer affected her so deeply that she was unable to cope with the possibility that she might have anything wrong. To her subconscious mind, it was all cancer. Now that she was awake and alert, she understood her instinctive reaction. When an individual has a nonbeneficial instinctual response, he or she will instinctively react in the same abnormal way until the injury is addressed and corrected. After the treatment was over, I asked her an important question or two.

Dr.: How do you feel?

Juanita: I feel better.

Dr.: Do you now understand why you reacted the way you did?

Juanita: Yes.

Dr.: From now on, is it necessary for you to react like you did prior to being treated?

Juanita: No, I believe I will be fine.

Dr.: Does it now affect you in any way if I bring up the subject of cancer, abnormal cells, or even the subject of surgery?

Juanita: No, it used to, but now I am okay. I don't have the uncontrollable urge to react to the word cancer anymore.

I saw her one week later and asked her if she was still okay in dealing with the subject of cancer. She replied that she was not affected by the subject. Three years later, she remained perfectly fine, completely unaffected by the fear of cancer.

# CHAPTER 12

## *The Brain That Refused To Allow Itself To Remember Any Memories Of The Past*

This chapter provides the insight that helps unravel the sensational prime time news stories concerning individuals who suddenly lose their memory. The common theme centers on a brain that refuses to allow itself to remember. There are many examples of such stories that make the headlines, such as the following.

A young man suddenly forgets who he is and has to learn to function in society once again. A middle aged healthy woman is found twenty miles from her home and does not remember her past or her family. A young girl experiences an illness and forgets how to walk in a forward direction but is able to walk backwards. A mother in her twenties does not recognize her husband or three children after she wakes up from surgery. Some individuals experience a traumatic event or injury that leads to the inability to remember anything. These people may appear as if they are in a zombie like state.

Although these stories attract great attention, they do not seem to end well. Frequently, there is no uniform effective treatment, and these individuals are left to hopefully regain their memory over time. Unfortunately, there is very little long term follow up because there is little reason to provide an update on a story unless there is a happy ending to report. This chapter seeks to unravel the mystery of how the brain clinically reacts to the challenges that it faces to prevent these spectacular losses of memory or amnesia.

Amnesia is a term commonly used to describe the loss of memory. When a person loses the ability to remember things that he or she should easily recall, it can have very severe consequences. This is especially true if the person who lost his memory has a significant responsibility to take care of or must provide financial support for the other members of his family. Many families are not prepared for the sudden change in their circumstances. These families will certainly struggle if the bread winner is unable to work because he has not only forgotten how to work, but how to drive to work as well. When these people seek medical care, they undergo an extensive workup which may include imaging and neurologic evaluation to make sure that an anatomical, metabolic, or structural cause of amnesia is not present. The list of possible illnesses that can lead to memory loss is fairly extensive. Such a list would include the common diagnosis of chronic alcohol abuse.

Not all memory loss can be treated successfully, but some forms of memory loss can be readily overcome. These are the types of memory loss that can occur when an individual experiences a loss of control leading to a nonstructural brain injury. A loss of control that leads to amnesia can occur when an individual is unable to cope with severe personal stress. Some of the medical terms used to describe this form of amnesia include dissociative fugue disorder, hysterical disorder, or even psychogenic amnesia. This form of amnesia or memory loss can result from severe emotional distress which can produce such a profound loss of control that a person can find himself in a zombie like or fugue state. This type of amnesia can result from the deliberate avoidance of unconscious or repressed memories. It is frequently triggered by the inability to handle a sudden overwhelmingly stressful challenge. Individuals who have suffered such insurmountable stress report that it is as if something in their brain just snapped and their memory suddenly went blank. This can result in a personal loss of identity, including the ability to remember the events or memories of the past. Fortunately, these affected individuals are able to recall recent events and are able to use new information that they experience to relearn some of their past. This may be the type of memory loss that describes someone you know or love. I would like to share with you the story of someone who suffered from this form of amnesia. I was able to help him overcome his amnesia in a single visit.

Lou is a thirty-two year-old otherwise healthy African American male who was found walking aimlessly down an interstate highway, in a trancelike state, at 4 a.m. A policeman thought that it was unusual for Lou to be walking around in the bitter cold without a jacket and stopped him to see if he was okay. When he was stopped by the police officer, Lou appeared to be in a zombie like state. The officer discovered that Lou could not remember who he was, why he was walking down the street in the middle the night, or any events of his past. When Lou was questioned by the officer, he simply drew a blank. He could not answer any personal questions about who he was or his past. He could not even remember the simplest of answers. Fortunately, he had identification in his wallet. He was taken to a local hospital and underwent imaging studies and a neurologic workup, all of which failed to show any impairment, injury, or obvious reason for his memory loss. He was given a diagnosis of amnesia and was taken home by his parents. His family was counseled that there was little that could be done. His family was also told that hopefully his memory would return over time. A month later, Lou was still unable to remember anything about his past. He had limited knowledge of how to take care of his needs and could not drive or work as he previously did in the welding trade. Lou's inability to work and provide support created a significant emotional and financial hardship for his family. He was referred to my office by his family doctor who had heard of my interest in helping such individuals.

When I saw him in my waiting room, he just sat there with a faceless expression and a catatonic blank stare. His eyes were fixed looking downward at the floor. This behavior is common in many patients with this form of memory loss. They have a persistent blank stare as if they are constantly searching for something that they lost. Lou just sat there in my office waiting to be seen, completely ignoring everything around him including, the television.

When I talked to Lou, he cautiously explained that he did not remember what had happened or the events that caused his amnesia or memory loss. Lou could not remember anything of his past. He was able to communicate to me in a slow conversant tone, but Lou could not remember anything or anyone prior to the date that he was found wandering.

In order to help Lou and similar individuals, it is important to recognize what the patient is actually suffering from. He apparently was doing well until something just snapped, and then his memory simply vanished and did not return. In this case, Lou's amnesia was caused by a nonstructural brain injury. This diagnosis is based on this patient's history, previous workup, and symptoms that he suffers from. Once this diagnosis is considered, the next step is to gain an understanding of how such an injury occurred. The pathway leading to the occurrence of this form of injury is listed below.

### How Insurmountable Emotional Distress Can Cause The Brain To Refuse To Allow Itself To Remember

Insurmountable emotional distress

Signals and challenges the nonstructural brain to respond to the distress so that a temporary state of loss of control occurs in the subconscious mind. This results in

Nonstructural brain confusion

This reflects the brain's ability to respond to and overcome the loss of control due to the symptoms or dysfunction caused by the insurmountable emotional distress.

The subconscious nonstructural brain is unable to resolve the profound loss of control.

↓

Instinctual imprinting then occurs

This results in some portions of the subconscious, nonstructural brain remaining in control and remaining unaltered and unaffected by the insurmountable emotional distress.

Other portions of the subconscious, nonstructural brain are overridden or reprogrammed by the process of instinctual imprinting. This leads to the formation of a…

Nonstructural brain injury

A nonstructural brain injury takes place due to the inability of the subconscious, nonstructural brain to resolve the loss of control and the subsequent negative instinctual imprinting that occurs due to the insurmountable emotional distress.

The result of this type of injury is that a nonbeneficial instinctual response is formed. From this point on, the portion of the subconscious mind that was injured will respond in an inappropriate way.

This type of injury may be clinically recognizable by the sudden profound memory loss that may include a fugue or zombie like state.

Once this form of brain injury is recognized, it can usually be successfully treated.

The principles of treatment are outlined below.

1. The first step to treating this patient's symptoms is to recognize that a nonstructural brain injury is present.

2. If such an injury is present, the memory loss that is experienced may be improved or eliminated by treatment.

3. Such treatment targets the portion of the nonstructural brain where the nonbeneficial instinctual responses producing the amnesia are occurring. The area where this injury is located is in the subconscious mind.

4. In order to be able to deal directly with and treat the subconscious mind, we have to be able to bypass the conscious thought process which prevents access to the subconscious mind.

5. A neuroreactive approach is appropriate in this case because of its profound ability to identify and remove the injured thought processes that negatively affect the nonstructural subconscious mind. This treatment should be able to eliminate the symptoms of memory loss or amnesia that are due to nonstructural brain injury and are not due to a metabolic or structural injury.

6. Once the nonbeneficial instinctual reactions are removed, memory instantly returns. Recurrent memory loss should not be expected unless the nonstructural brain is subjected to a separate loss of control in the future.

During treatment, Lou was initially unable to verbally communicate with me. The reason for this inability was that the issue surrounding his memory loss was so disturbing to him that he was prevented from verbalizing it out loud. His lips moved, yet no words emerged. As a result of treatment, he was able to overcome the insurmountable loss of control that led to the development of his amnesia. He was finally able to verbally talk about the events that led to the amnesia because those events became only memories that had absolutely no effect on his ability to maintain control. Once the nonstructural injury was treated, there was nothing preventing Lou from using his memory.

**Lou's memory was present the entire time he experienced amnesia. It's just that Lou could not consciously retrieve these**

**memories. The portion of Lou's nonstructural brain that was injured prevented access to those memories.**

Immediately after treatment, his memory completely returned. Lou had complete recall of all the events, people, places, and memories of his past. His memory was all there, just as it was before he lost control. He could think clearly once again.

His spouse was brought into the room and was in a state of disbelief that her husband who had seen so many specialists was able to once again have a normal memory. She proceeded to quiz, question, and test his recall until she was sure that he was indeed cured. Once she realized that her husband had regained his memory, she was able to experience overwhelming joy.

# CHAPTER 13

*The Brain That Refused To Allow*
*The Body To Lose Weight*

This chapter explores how the inability to lose weight and keep it off is frequently related to the presence of an underlying nonstructural injury. This is a silent injury that sabotages many individuals' conscious efforts to be in control of themselves, their bodies, and their weight. This chapter also provides valuable insight as to why gastric bypass surgery alone may not achieve the long term results that people are led to believe that the procedure holds for them. The explanations provided will allow many to discover one of the missing pieces that prevents individuals from losing weight and keeping it off. This includes an understanding of a brain that refuses to allow itself to lose weight. Many of the people presented in this chapter may strike you as similar to someone you know who has these difficulties. One such person is a woman named Annie.

Annie suffered her entire life from being overweight. She could not lose any significant amount of weight no matter what she did. She tried numerous diets, weight loss programs, and gimmicks on TV. She also read all the popular diet books without success. She failed to lose any weight, so she tried various exercise programs as best she could. Her weight of 285 pounds caused her blood pressure and blood sugars to increase to the point of her needing medication. She eventually decided that she needed additional help and sought advice concerning gastric bypass surgery. While preparing for gastric bypass surgery, she saw a dietitian as well as a psychiatrist who felt that she was a suitable candidate for the procedure. She finally underwent the procedure. She did well and started to lose weight. She went from 285 pounds to 160 pounds over the course of one year. She noticed that her diabetes and hypertension vanished as soon as she lost her first ninety pounds. She was also quite happy with her appearance and the newfound attention she was receiving. Her surgeon was happy as well. As the next two years passed, she started regaining the weight that she had initially lost. When I saw her, she weighed 219 pounds, which was a weight gain of fifty-nine pounds from her lowest point. Her diabetes and high blood pressure had also returned. I asked her why she was experiencing such a weight gain when she was previously doing quite well. She said that she did not know.

This is a very common occurrence in individuals who undergo gastric bypass surgery. This scenario also occurs in people who diet, exercise, and achieve success in the short-term, but eventually gain back all the weight that they lost. Such individuals initially do quite well and lose a considerable amount of weight. The medical community views this as an overwhelming success. After all, this person underwent a surgery and lost a lot of weight. This "success" leads to the following question, "If bariatric surgery or dieting is so successful, why are so many people unable to maintain their weight loss year after year?"

Many good reasons and excuses can be put forth to explain rebound weight gain. I have always felt that it is occurring because something is missing or is not being addressed. This observation has more to do with the process involved in preparing an individual for the upcoming surgical procedure or the future anticipated diet. The patients who I have seen all report that they get dietary counseling, take classes, attend support groups, and are monitored for  suitability to undergo a gastric bypass procedure. They even see a psychiatrist who works with the weight-loss surgeon. The psychiatrist's role is to determine if this patient is psychologically and emotionally prepared undergo the surgery and handle the changes that may occur after the surgery.

## Eating For Comfort

If all this preparation is provided, what can possibly be missing. This same question has been repeated over and over again by a large number of people who I've talked to over several years. When I ask these individuals why they didn't keep the weight off, I get the predictable answers. These range from "I don't know" to blaming their failure on some form of stress or difficulty. Most caregivers take these answers at face value and reply that these individuals need to stick to their diets, choose their foods wisely, and exercise. Those who have had gastric bypass surgery or have tried the diet of the week know that this answer will not work. If this solution was effective then these individuals would have consciously done so without needing to be told. This line of questioning needs to be more specific in order to arrive at the reason why so many people experience rebound weight gain. When the same question is asked in a different manner, many practitioners and individuals can arrive closer to the truth, which is more difficult to talk about. Let us see what happened when I discussed this subject with Annie.

**Physician:** Many people find that they eat because deep inside they feel a certain amount of comfort when they do so. These individuals don't even realize that they are eating to feel comfortable. Many people eat in order to distract themselves whenever they think of an unpleasant thought, event, or disturbing past memory. Annie, I want you to think back now. When you find yourself eating to feel comfortable, are you doing so because you're responding to an unpleasant thought or experience?

**Annie** looks at the physician with a defensive look....A moment later she responds.

**Annie:** I don't know.

**Physician:** Be honest with me (looking directly at Annie). When you think of something that is disturbing, you find yourself feeling the urge to eat, don't you?

**Annie:** (Pauses)…Yes

**Physician:** When you think about it, you know exactly what thought it is because this thought occurs so frequently it causes you to eat when you do not need to. The same thought also prevents you from losing weight.

**Annie:** (after a another pause)…Yes

**Physician:** I want you to tell me what event, memory, or thought in your past is disturbing you and causing you to eat uncontrollably.

**Annie:** I…..

At this point, the patient usually realizes that the physician is serious about helping her and that the superficial deception will not work anymore. I've also found that these individuals may or may not consciously be able to tell me exactly what the unpleasant past memory or experience is that they are trying to repress through eating for comfort. If a person cannot tell you the exact details, then he and she usually will be able to narrow it down to a person, an event, or a time period when the individual was under great stress and then lost control.

### The Weight Loss Game Of Give And Take

Most caregivers may not ask these questions because it may involve a time commitment as well as a certain amount of discomfort on the part of the caregiver. This uneasiness exists because many caregivers experience difficulty attempting to help a patient overcome deep emotional and dysfunctional issues. These caregivers may feel very uncomfortable to simply arrive at the source of their patient's dysfunction without being able to offer a way to overcome it. When we deal with the deep underlying reasons why people eat for comfort in order to forget or to repress memories, there is a trade-off or an unwritten deal that is being communicated. The deal is that the patient will be honest and tell the hidden truth, but in return for the truth, the patient expects the physician to make him or her better. Since many caregivers may not have been trained to address this challenge, they simply accept the patient's answer, "I don't know" or it was simply "stress" that prevented him or her from keeping the weight off. This unwritten interaction between caregiver and patient is a form of the game of "give-and-take." The patient will give the caregiver the superficial excuse of "stress" or "I don't know," and the caregiver will respond to this answer by saying "stick to the diet, limit portion size, and exercise." In this way, patients do not have to divulge their past which they want to repress, and the caregiver does not have to feel uncomfortable by uncovering something that he or she may not be able to successfully address. These challenging personal issues are frequently understood as a "psych" issue so that a timely referral is suggested but never acted on by the patient. The reason that they do not act on this recommendation is that most patients may not have the financial resources to cover psychiatric services for weight loss. In addition, many patients simply do not want to initiate a process in which the answer lies in multiple office visits over a long period of time. Another reason that patients do not seek help is that they do not want to be labeled as someone with a "psychological issue."

In order to understand why many individuals are unable to achieve a long-term weight loss despite diet, exercise, and bariatric surgery, we need to consider that a nonstructural brain injury may be present. The following pathway provides significant insight as to how the brain can undergo injury that results in its refusal to allow the body to maintain weight loss.

**How a nonstructural brain injury can produce a loss of control which progresses into an uncontrollable urge to eat:**

We start out being good enough and in control

↓

Unfortunately, we may experience a potential emotional or interactive injury.

These commonly include family issues, abuse, and molestation.

This signals and challenges the brain to respond to the injury so that a state of loss of control occurs. This is termed...

Nonstructural brain confusion

This is the brain's ability to respond to and overcome the loss of control by understanding what went wrong, being able to adapt, learning from one's mistakes, correcting any mistakes, doing better next time, and remaining good enough not to be affected by the potential emotional and interactive injury.

Despite treatment, the subconscious, nonstructural brain is unable to completely resolve this loss of control. When this happens...

Instinctual imprinting occurs.

This results in some portions of the nonstructural subconscious brain remaining in control and remaining unaltered and unaffected by the emotional or interactive injury.

Other portions of the subconscious, nonstructural brain are overridden or reprogrammed by the process of instinctual imprinting. This leads to the formation of a...

Nonstructural brain injury

A nonstructural brain injury results from the inability of the subconscious, nonstructural brain to resolve the loss of control and the subsequent negative instinctual imprinting that occurs.

The result of this type of injury is that a nonbeneficial instinctual response is formed. From this point on, the portion of the subconscious mind that was injured will continually respond in an inappropriate way.

↓

This type of injury may be clinically recognizable by the unconscious or instinctual urge to find comfort in eating in order to distract oneself or "forget" whenever one thinks of an unpleasant thought, event, or disturbing memory. This can express itself as uncontrollable weight gain, rebound weight gain, failing to respond to diet and exercise, binge eating, and a host of other dysfunctions.

↓

Once a nonbeneficial instinctual response is recognized, it can usually be successfully treated.

### Avoiding The Stumbling Blocks

This explanation can explain why so many individuals regain their lost weight after dieting or gastric bypass surgery. The failure to maintain weight loss despite diet and surgery is similar to leaving stumbling blocks before a blind person. When a series of stumbling blocks is placed before someone who cannot see, it is only a matter of time before the blind person falls.

Successful long-term results can be achieved once the stumbling blocks or the instinctual responses that do not benefit an individual are removed. This is done through the understanding that the causative injury is occurring in the nonstructural brain. When we casually talk to these individuals, we are essentially talking to their conscious minds. In order to be effective, we need to bypass the conscious thought process. When this is done, we can effectively correct the person's underlying nonbeneficial instinctual responses. This will eliminate the need for an individual to continue to unconsciously react to his or her past by eating to forget in order to feel comfortable. This treatment approach can enable someone to be successful in the present as well as the future because the stumbling blocks of the past have been removed. Many times, all that is needed is a single visit. This approach makes much more sense than simply relying on diet, exercise, and/or gastric bypass surgery.

### Conflicts Of Interest

Another issue that contributes to long term failure and rebound weight gain is the relationship between patients seeking bypass surgery and their caregivers. Many individuals undergoing gastric bypass surgery are required to see a psychiatrist. The psychiatrist is supposed to identify whether or not this patient is a suitable candidate for undergoing the gastric bypass procedure. Unfortunately, there can be many conflicts of interest inherent in the process of pre-operative evaluation and treatment. The first conflict of interest deals with the relationship between the surgeon and a particular psychiatrist. The surgeon will usually send a potential bypass patient to a specific psychiatrist for presurgical clearance. During this visit, the patient is evaluated to determine the patient's mental and emotional stability. There is an unwritten and usually unspoken understanding that unless something is significantly wrong with this individual, the patient will be cleared for surgery. Surgeons monitor their patients quite closely. Since the surgeon strongly believes that his potential patient would be an excellent candidate and would deeply benefit from the surgery, the surgeon will not be very pleased when his patient is unable to get a psychiatric clearance. When this occurs too often, the surgeon's answer will be to find another psychiatrist who will be willing to understand that potential gastric bypass patients need to be cleared to undergo the surgical procedure.

Patients also contribute significantly to their under treatment preoperatively. They usually do not volunteer the deep, underlying reasons why they instinctively eat in order to feel comfortable as well as to forget. They almost universally respond that they if they were to bring up their deep and painful emotional issues, they would run the risk of not being considered an appropriate surgical candidate.

They feel that they would be viewed as "crazy" or a "psych" case and would not be allowed to undergo the surgical procedure.

The same is true concerning many diet centers and weight loss programs that stress calorie counting, limiting portions, and exercise. While these programs are able to help educate as well as promote healthy lifestyle habits, many of these programs or popular diets have much more difficulty achieving lasting long-term results. One reason is that they only deal with a person's conscious thought process and fail to adequately address the underlying issues hidden deep inside that are present subconsciously.

## Clinically Speaking

Annie finally told me in a sad tone of voice that her uncontrollable need to eat was due to an event that took place in her childhood. It was difficult for her to understand the details of this memory. Annie was uncomfortable and a little tearful even trying to think about it. Once the influence of the conscious thought process was eliminated, Annie was able to recall the event that led to the formation of her nonstructural brain injury.

She related that as a young child she had a close family member who suffered from severe anorexia and was wasting away. Along with her mother and her sister, she happened to visit this person just hours before this individual's death. While waiting for her mother in the next room, she overheard her mother telling her sister, "See what happens when you starve yourself. I really hope you do not allow this to happen to you." Apparently, Annie was deeply affected by her mother's words. She was so overwhelmed by the death of her family member that she experienced a loss of control that led to the formation of a nonbeneficial instinctual reaction. This nonstructural injury was characterized by eating for comfort as a way of inappropriately responding to the thought of this unpleasant memory. Annie was unconsciously and instinctively eating to forget.

Once Annie was able to understand how her brain reacted to what had occurred, she found that it was unnecessary to abnormally react to this event through inappropriate eating. She was able to regain control of her weight. I saw her yearly for the next two years and she was quite happy. She continued to have no difficulty controlling her urge to eat. Clinically, her weight stayed consistent at 167 pounds, which is a significant long term weight loss from her prior weight of 285 pounds. Her diabetes and high blood pressure were not present anymore as well.

### Additional Clinical Insight

The following presentations highlight how sensitive the subconscious thought process is to emotional or interactive injury. Such injuries can lead to a brain that refuses to allow the body to lose weight or maintain weight loss. **This is especially true when rape or molestation is involved.** These traumatic injuries need to be addressed in a timely manner to avoid a lifetime of dysfunction characterized by ongoing nonbeneficial instinctual responses. Unfortunately, few cases of these traumatic injuries are clinically recognized and effectively treated so that the affected individuals can regain their ability to be in control.

### Chemotherapy Causing Weight Dysfunction

Sally was in her late thirties when she underwent surgery followed by chemotherapy for ovarian cancer. Her chemotherapy was quite aggressive. As a result, she experienced ongoing nausea and vomiting that prevented her ability to maintain her weight. Over the course of the chemotherapy, she experienced a very significant weight loss and was frequently hospitalized to treat her recurrent dehydration. I saw her nine months after she was discharged from the hospital and had finished all of her chemotherapy. Sally related she was finally able to eat once more and had no feelings of nausea and vomiting. She also found that a new issue had surfaced. She stated that she was gaining weight excessively due to an uncontrollable urge to eat. She said she knew that she should not be eating the way that she was bingeing.

She claimed that she felt powerless to fight the continual urge to eat. Sally claimed that she just couldn't help it. I asked her if anything had occurred in her past that would cause her to have this uncontrollable urge. Sally said that she could not consciously remember anything that would cause her to continually eat and gain an excessive amount of weight.

During treatment, Sally was able to recall overhearing her surgeon talking to the nurse outside her room. She remembered that the surgeon was whispering to the nurse, but in spite of this Sally could hear everything that was said. Her doctor was telling the nurse that unless Sally started to gain a considerable amount of weight, she may not be strong enough to overcome her illness. He was deeply worried that he would have to stop her chemotherapy before this treatment had a chance to effectively remove all her remaining cancer. These words deeply affected Sally so that she experienced a profound loss of control, resulting in the negative imprinting of her subconscious mind. This led to the formation of a nonbeneficial instinctual response characterized by the uncontrollable urge to eat excessively. This urge continued long after she had recovered from her cancer. Her compulsion to eat was now making her significantly overweight and posing a serious risk to her future health. Once the underlying nonbeneficial instinctual response was eliminated, Sally found it unnecessary to respond to a past event that was negatively affecting her present and future health. The result of this was that Sally was able to effectively control her eating habits and slim down to an appropriate and very healthy weight.

## Rape, Molestation, and Weight Dysfunction

The story of this next patient is the story of so many individuals that I see in clinical practice. Zoe is a twenty-three year old female who was seen in my office for a yearly examination. I noticed that Zoe had been steadily gaining weight with every yearly visit, but it seemed that this year she was having a very difficult time controlling her weight. She had gone from 146 pounds two years earlier to 186 pounds, with a large amount of that weight gain occurring in the last year. I asked her if there was a reason for this weight gain. She replied with the typical answer of "stress." I then asked her what kind of stress would cause her to completely lose control and gain such a large amount of weight in just one year. She cited some seemingly minor incidents in her life but nothing that would be significant enough to cause her to gain so much weight. I then asked Zoe if her ability to control her weight was getting worse each day. She replied that it was. I informed Zoe that many people find that they eat because deep inside they feel a certain amount of comfort when they do so. Many times these individuals don't even realize that they are eating to feel comfortable. In reality, many people tend to eat in order to distract themselves as a nonbeneficial instinctual response whenever they think of an unpleasant thought, event, or disturbing memory. I told Zoe to think back to when she feels the urge to eat to feel comfortable. I then asked her if she was doing so because she was responding to an unpleasant thought or experience. The sad look on her face and the pain in her eyes told me that the answer was yes. I told her to be very honest with me so that I could attempt to help her. I then asked her the question that required an answer deeply buried inside that affected her on a daily basis. **"Zoe, have you ever been molested or raped in the past?"** This question had a profound effect on her. The tears started flowing as she replied, "Yes."

Zoe said that she was five years old when a close family member molested her over and over again until she was seven years old. She said that she was only a child and did not know any better. Since that time, she has been so ashamed and embarrassed that she has never mentioned this abuse to anyone but her mother. When she confided in her mother, she was just told not to tell anyone or else child protective services would take her away. She was very sad that her mother did not do more to help her. I asked Zoe if this disturbing incident of her past causes her to feel the urge to eat when she is not hungry. I also questioned her to see if the same thoughts also prevented her from losing weight. She replied yes to both.

This individual appears to have experienced a loss of control that resulted in a nonstructural brain injury. This led to the formation of a nonbeneficial instinctual response with symptoms that include uncontrollable eating, excessive weight gain, and the inability to effectively lose weight. Zoe was stuck instinctively reacting to her past every time she recalled those disturbing thoughts. She was unconsciously eating for comfort as a way to repress to these unpleasant memories, events, or experiences. Zoe was essentially **eating to forget**.

Zoe's unpleasant history is not unique. I frequently encounter the scenario of how rape and molestation lead to nonstructural issues, including weight gain. It is also important to emphasize that the person responsible for these molestations frequently appears as someone who is well known to the victim. This may include a close friend, boyfriend of the mother, or family member. It is less likely that a perfect stranger magically appears and molests someone.

Now let's explore how we can enable those who suffer like Zoe to overcome the effects of molestation in order to allow them to finally heal and get better. One way to achieve this is to use a neuroreactive approach. I informed Zoe that I could help her regain control so that she would not have to eat for comfort or experience the need to instinctually react to her past memories of rape and molestation. I told her that she will always have the ability to remember her past, but her past would have absolutely no effect on her. All her past would be is a memory and nothing more. This is what can be accomplished when we remove the underlying nonstructural injury that prevents a person from achieving long term control of their weight and emotional well being.

I was able to help Zoe overcome the difficulties of her past that negatively affected her present and caused her ongoing weight issues. Once the nonstructural injury had been successfully corrected, she found it unnecessary to eat to forget. Her prior molestation did not affect her well being anymore. Zoe was finally able to regain the control that she had lost a very long time ago. She was very pleased that she was able to lose weight, but she was even happier that she was able to maintain the weight loss. Two years later she weighed in at a thin 138 pounds.

# CHAPTER 14

*The Brain That Refused To Allow Itself To Go To The Dentist*

One improvement that people really appreciate in their lives is the ability to go to the dentist's office without suffering from any type of mental or physical trauma. Dental fear is frequently related to the actual or perceived memories of your past.

### The Challenge Of Undergoing A Dental Procedure

Just think about what is happening inside your mind the whole time that dental "work" is occurring. You have to sit in a chair with your mouth wide open. There is nothing else you can do while at the mercy of the person working on your teeth. While this is occurring, you will experience various sensations. Some of them may be painful, while others will be perceived as even more traumatic. These sensations bombard the nerve endings that signal each of your five senses. The other thing that takes place is time distortion; even a few minutes seem to last a lifetime. In summary, you're placing yourself in a situation in which the brain is deeply challenged to remain in control. These events can lead to a brain that refuses to allow itself to go to the dentist.

This scenario fits quite nicely into our model of loss of control, nonstructural brain injury, and the brain's inability to recover from perceived dramatic injury. By being knowledgeable of the sequence of events that lead to this type of loss of control, you can gain an understanding of how to prevent a loss of control from occurring and how to treat a person who has undergone dental trauma. Let us now look at the events that take place at a dentist's office that can lead to the development of a nonstructural brain injury.

### How A Nonstructural Dental Injury Can Develop

Visiting the dentist or undergoing a dental procedure

↓

Can produce physical, psychological, and emotional injury as well as…

Perceived olfactory injury,

Perceived auditory injury from instruments, that make sounds which the brain associates with pain, or from inappropriate verbalizations from the dental staff.

Perceived visual injury due to seeing the procedure, the drill, and sharp instruments as they enter your mouth.

Perceived taste injury, including the taste of medicine, anesthetic, blood, and different resins.

Perceived sensory injury due to pain involving the teeth, gums, lips, tongue, and nerves. Additional long-term pain may also occur at the temporal mandibular joint (TMJ).

Time distortion

Being unable to anticipate what is coming next:

This signals and challenges the nonstructural brain to respond to the perceived injury so that a state of loss of control occurs in the subconscious mind. This results in

Nonstructural brain confusion.

This is the brain's ability to respond to or overcome the loss of control due to the symptoms or dysfunction from the dental visit or dental procedure.

↓

Despite treatment, the subconscious, nonstructural brain is unable to completely resolve the loss of control. This possibly occurs because you are stuck in the chair with your mouth open and cannot move. This can lead to accepting these perceived injuries as actual injuries. This results in ...

↓

Instinctual imprinting

This results in some portions of the subconscious, nonstructural brain remaining in control and remaining unaltered and unaffected by the dental visit or dental procedure.

Other portions of the subconscious, nonstructural brain are now overridden or reprogrammed by the process of instinctual imprinting. This leads to the formation of a...

↓

Nonstructural brain injury

A nonstructural brain injury occurs due to the inability of the subconscious, nonstructural brain to resolve the loss of control and the subsequent negative instinctual imprinting that occurs due to the symptoms, injury, or dysfunction caused by the dental visit or dental procedure.

↓

This type of injury is easily recognizable by the abnormal or undesirable side effects, physical symptoms, or behavioral changes that remain long after the individual has "recovered" from the dental experience. When this occurs, people may experience nonbeneficial instinctual behaviors of pain, avoidance, loss of control, phobias, anxiety, fear, and even panic.

This same pathway can be used to prevent such an injury from occurring in the first place by making it unnecessary for the person to experience any type of occurrence that would lead to a loss of control.

When the subconscious mind is prepared to instinctively respond in a way that will benefit an individual prior to undergoing a dental procedure, the outcome is remarkably different. The brain is able to stay in control and does not accept the signals and challenges from the site of injury. The brain has understood that these potential challenges leading to a loss of control would be present at the time of the dental visit. The brain has anticipated how to instinctually answer these potential challenges. When the brain has been enabled to respond instinctually, the brain does not have to succumb to the realistic risk of losing control through conscious thinking. It is when conscious thought is bypassed that one is able to respond instinctually. An individual will be able to maintain a relaxed state and will find it unnecessary to experience pain, discomfort, or emotional trauma. This leads to the ability to successfully undergo the dental procedure as well as achieve a speedier and more pleasant visit without discomfort. The reason that no pain or injury occurs is because the brain has been preconditioned to instinctually maintain control so it will not accept the signals of perceived injury. This is consistent with the neuroreactive principle that an individual only feels pain and injury when the brain allows him or her to feel pain and injury.

It is possible to give ordinary individuals the ability to make dental procedures a pain free experience. These are a few examples of how this can make a difference in a person's life.

**Root Canal Pain**

Lindsay came to my office one morning for an evaluation of a condition involving an ovarian cyst seen on an ultrasound. After the evaluation, the patient complained about extreme pain coming from her right lower jaw. She related that she had undergone a dental procedure prior to seeing me in the office. She said that she had root canal surgery performed in two teeth, and the pain was getting unbearable.

She rated it a ten out of ten. While she was sitting on my examination table, I made a seemingly impossible statement. I said to her that I could get rid of her pain in only a few minutes by retraining how the nonstructural brain to responds to pain. I told her I only needed to talk to her, and all she needed to do was to be a good listener and her pain would be completely gone.  I also mentioned that once the pain was gone, it would stay gone forever.  Since she felt that her pain could not be much worse, she was quite receptive to having her pain go away. Immediately after treatment, she noticed that the pain was not there. The root canal pain had vanished.  Lindsay was amazed and even went looking for the pain by biting down, poking, and prodding the area where those two teeth had been.  To her amazement, the pain was completely gone.

In a kind gesture of appreciation, she asked me to marry her, and the offer included a four year old child as well. Instant family! I deeply appreciated this gesture since no one had ever asked me to marry her in my entire life.  At a follow up visit, Lindsay reported that the pain had not bothered her again.

It is important to note that another painful condition known as "Dry Socket" is also easily and effectively treated using a neuroreactive approach.

**Another example**

One day when I was rounding in the hospital, I encountered a registered nurse named Sheila who was taking care of a patient of mine.  After inquiring how my patient was doing that day, I asked her how she was doing.  She mentioned that she was going to undergo a root canal in the near future. She was deeply worried about the pain that she would experience. I told her that it was unnecessary to experience pain when she gets the procedure done and, since she took such good care of my patient, I would give her the ability to be completely comfortable when she underwent the procedure. After a brief treatment, Sheila discovered that she had a newfound ability.  This ability enabled her to make her entire mouth and gums so numb that she was unable to feel a needle pushing deeply into her gums. Furthermore, she was even able to demonstrate this newfound ability to a crowd of nurses at the nearby nursing station. Everyone was deeply impressed. She thanked me and said to me, "Will you marry me?" I was quite intrigued. I had received two marriage proposals in fewer than two weeks. I always thought that you had to get to know a person or at least go on a few dates before someone proposed. What I learned is all you have to do is give the gift of dental anesthesia and you can instantly be viewed as "a keeper." If only I had known this when I was much younger and single.

Another patient, Darlene, was in the office to see me for a gynecological matter just prior to her appointment with her dentist for a tooth extraction. Since I had given her the ability to create anesthesia for another medical condition, I reminded her that she could use that ability to also make her mouth so numb that she would not require any anesthesia for the extraction. I told her to make that area of her mouth completely numb using the instructions I had previously given her. She did so and said that the area was now numb. I asked her how numb it was? She replied that it was very numb. So I got a needle and deeply probed the area. I found it to be completely numb, just like she said it was. I told her to give me a call and let me know what her dentist's reaction was. She called me and let me know that she did not require any anesthesia to get her tooth extracted. She said that the dentist found it to be unbelievable that she had such pain control. She underwent the procedure in a completely painless manner, and when she was offered pain medication after the procedure to take home, she said it was completely unnecessary. She kindly thanked me. This patient essentially underwent and recovered from the procedure before the procedure was actually performed.

These are some of the possibilities that can occur when an effective form of treatment is used to make it unnecessary to experience any discomfort or pain in a patient who will be completely awake while undergoing a dental procedure.

# CHAPTER 15

*Legal Implications That May Result From A Brain That
Refuses To Allow Itself To Get Better*

Accidents happen. When they occur, we all do our best to heal from the injury. In our present society, we believe there must be some-one to blame when an accident occurs that leaves a person unable to fully recover. Legally, we have the right to blame other people for complications resulting from an accident, injury, or medical treatment. If we can convince a jury that we have experienced pain, disability, or suffering due to the fault of another, then we may be entitled to collect monetary damages. In many cases, the formula goes some-thing like this.

As a result of the behavior of the guilty party, I experienced an acci-dent, injury, or medical complication, and I was unable to get better. Since that event, I continue to experience pain, disability, and suffer-ing. I have been unable to _____, which has directly resulted in a personal, financial, or emotional loss. Thus, I will sue for damages because I did not get better. I will link the injuries that I have to the doctor who performed the procedure or the person who I believe is the cause of my injury.

**Until now, it is assumed that the injury was a result of some-thing that the doctor did wrong since the person was fine before the procedure.**

Up to this time, it had not been possible in many cases to show that an injury was unrelated to surgery or medical treatment. We just assume that the surgeon who performed the surgery was the direct cause of the injury and is guilty because of the way the patient recovered. This recovery included the symptoms of a new onset injury or disability.

The question arises, "What if the surgeon did not do anything wrong, but the patient still did not recover the way that he or she was expected to?" Let us take a look and see how this applies to the diagnosis of nonstuctural injury.

Imagine a patient who has undergone surgery in the area of her groin to remove a fatty tumor. Since the tumor was pretty deep and located near many of the nerves that innervate her leg, it became quite challenging to remove the tumor. After the surgery, the patient experienced numbness in some areas of her upper leg, along with pain, including pins and needles sensations in other areas. She also noticed that her leg had lost the ability to move as it once did and she could not ambulate normally. This patient underwent the usual diagnostic workups as well as treatments of medication, injections, physical therapy, and time for the area to heal. Unfortunately, her leg did not get much better, so this patient had to live with the pain, suffering, and disability.

When we view this patient from a legal standpoint:

1. This patient underwent surgery.

2. This patient obviously experienced an injury at the time of surgery.

3. This patient did not recover and continues to experience pain, suffering, and disability as well as the inability to work in her profession.

4. The surgeon is to blame for the patient's injury.

Thus, the patient can sue the surgeon and possibly collect a lot of money.

All that needs to happen is for the jury to be convinced that the surgeon must have caused the injury since the injury was not present prior to the surgery. This sounds like a slam dunk for an even not so good attorney. This is what frequently happens using our present knowledge of how medicine or surgery can affect an individual.

Now let's consider a scenario in which the surgeon did nothing wrong and was not responsible for causing the patient's injury. This approach is quite valid. When we consider the clinical evidence presented in this book, we gain the new understanding that similar injury or complications may actually be due to a nonstructural injury.

### How Surgery Produces A Nonstructural Injury

Surgery is performed which produces an injury

This signals and challenges the nonstructural brain to respond to the injury so that a temporary state of loss of control occurs in the subconscious mind. This results in

Nonstructural brain confusion.

This reflects the brain's ability to respond to and overcome the loss of control due to the symptoms or dysfunction caused by the surgery.

Despite treatment, the subconscious, nonstructural brain is unable to completely resolve the loss of control.

Instinctual imprinting occurs

This results in some portions of the subconscious, nonstructural brain remaining in control and remaining unaltered and unaffected by the surgery.

Other portions of the subconscious, nonstructural brain are now over-ridden or reprogrammed by the process of instinctual imprinting. This leads to the formation of a…

↓

Nonstructural brain injury.

A nonstructural brain injury occurs due to the inability of the subcon-scious, nonstructural brain to resolve the loss of control and the subse-quent negative instinctual imprinting that occurs.

↓

The result of this type of injury is that a nonbeneficial instinctual response is formed. From this point on, the portion of the subcon-scious mind that was injured will respond in an inappropriate way.

↓

These responses may include partial recovery, pain, hypersensitivity, hyposensitivity, loss of function, decreased range of motion, decreased mobility, numbness, pins and needle sensations, sensitivity to pres-sure, emotional, psychological, or neurological dysfunction, weakness, achy muscles, or rigidity.

When we use the pathway that shows how nonstructural injury occurs due to surgery, we can see that it is not so clear that the surgeon has committed any type of malpractice or caused injury. To under-stand this point using the above pathway, let's look at the events once more:

1. This patient underwent surgery. A surgery is a type of injury to a specific area of the body.

2. At the time of surgery, this patient experienced an injury at a specific area that is at the site of the surgical incision. This is the area where the actual surgery took place. Since the surgery, the patient has subsequently recovered physically from the injury

experienced at the specific area where the surgery actually took place.

3. In addition, the whole experience of being operated on was perceived by the nonstructural brain as an overwhelming challenge that led to the patient experiencing a loss of control. This loss of control was unable to be properly resolved by the nonstructural subconscious brain. This led to a portion of the subconscious brain becoming negatively imprinted, which resulted in the formation of a nonstructural brain injury.

4. Since a portion of the nonstructural brain was unable to fully recover, a nonbeneficial instinctual response emerged with the symptoms of pain, suffering, and disability.

5. Therefore, no injury occurred at the site of surgery where the actual operation was performed. The actual ongoing symptomatic injury occurred in the nonstructural subconscious brain. The surgeon is not able to predict nor is he or she responsible for how a portion of a person's nonstructural brain responds to a potential loss of control. This includes the surgical procedure that the patient had undergone.

## What is the clinical evidence for a neuroreactive injury?

If such an injury was responsible for this individual's symptoms of pain, sensations of pins and needles, numbness, and loss of range of motion, then it would be reasonable that the symptoms would permanently resolve after treatment.

The clinical evidence is that this individual's symptoms of pain, sensations of pins and needles, numbness, and loss of range of motion were reversed using a neuroreactive approach. This treatment enabled this person's subconscious memory to overcome the nonstructural injury and regain control. Three years of pain and suffering and disability were reversed in under fifteen minutes.

**A contemporary understanding of the formation of nonstructural injury can not only help many who suffer get better, but may also prevent many individuals from facing legal challenges from injuries for which they were not responsible.**

When people are able to overcome illness and get better, it is a good thing. It is also good not to face legal challenges for things that are beyond our control. Thus, it is important to attempt to see if a person's symptoms can be identified as consistent with a nonstructural injury. If a person's symptoms are consistent with such an injury, it is possible that this injury can be successfully treated and easily overcome.

**The diagnosis of a nonstructural brain injury and its successful treatment can be used to help a great many people who suffer, but there are also considerable concerns that this diagnosis can be abused by individuals who seek a monetary reward.**

When treatment has been attempted on a greedy individual or a person who may expect a big payout, this individual may be faced with the following choice: does he or she desire the monetary reward or does this individual want to overcome the disability and feel better. There may be a less than honest person who, despite overcoming the injury, continues to act as though he or she is still injured in order to get the monetary reward. This is a challenge that must be faced and addressed by the legal community.

# CHAPTER 16

*The Brain That Allowed Itself To Heal By
Responding To Placebos*

Most people have probably heard a news story or two about a phenomenon called the placebo effect. These news stories usually explore the beneficial effects of placebos. Placebos are pills containing essentially nothing but sugar. They are reported to make people better or enable them to overcome the symptoms they suffer from. We are amazed when we hear these stories because it challenges us to think that a trip to the candy store is all that it would take to get better. There have been many explanations that have been put forth to try to unravel the mystery of how placebos work. Unfortunately, these theories usually fall short of allowing us to understand what is really occurring, so we use the vague term "the placebo effect."

When we deconstruct what a placebo is made of, we discover that it is made of essentially nothing but a gelatin capsule filled with sugar. There is nothing in it that would allow us to get better and overcome what ails us. Yet it seems that when we give placebos to individuals, there is a statistically significant percentage of people who improve or get better. This challenges the way we think about things. When we accept that placebos work, we are also accepting the idea that when we use a placebo, we are creating something (an improvement or a cure) out of nothing.

## A Typical Placebo Experiment

Placebos are also the gold standard by which we are able to study things in medicine in order to determine if a treatment or cure is better than random luck or chance. In medicine, we use what is termed a double blind study. These studies are comparisons between a specific drug treatment and what occurs when nothing is done. A hypothetical example of such a study would be to treat 1000 individuals with similar headache symptoms with a new medication that can improve or cure them. Of these 1000 individuals, 500 would randomly be given sugar pills or placebos. The other 500 random individuals would receive pills that could potentially help remove their recurrent headaches. There would be no way for the 1000 individuals receiving pills to know if they took a real pill or a placebo. After a specified period of time, the study's participants would be questioned to determine how many individuals in each group improved. The goal of such a study is twofold. The first is to determine if the new drug really worked and improved the participant's headaches. The second goal is to show that it improved a person's headaches in a statistically better way than the group taking just a placebo.

In the business world, a "valid" successful study can make a company billions in profits, and failure can result in a "migraine." There is a lot at stake, especially for companies that create new medications. The underlying assumption of these studies is that something is being compared to nothing. Perhaps this is an incorrect assumption. What if it were possible to explain the "nothing" and show that a placebo is really something that is not difficult to understand.

### Applying Neuroreactive Thinking

When we apply the neuroreactive approach to the question of how a placebo works, things get much clearer. Using this approach, we start out with the same simple scenario in which a person took a sugar pill and got better. Was there anything that was contained in the pill that allowed a person to get better? The answer is no. Did the sugar pill change a person's internal chemistry so that he or she improved? The answer is also no. So what is it that a placebo is doing that allows a person to get better? The answer is that a placebo is a simplistic way to attempt to bypass the conscious thought process in order to directly treat an underlying nonstructural brain injury. It is this injury that may be responsible for the symptoms that we experience.

Our understanding of placebos changes when we realize that placebos are actually targeting and treating something. This makes sense because our knowledge of the neuroreactive principles states that:

1. In most illnesses, physical traumas, and emotional dysfunctions, there are two injuries: an actual structural one and a nonstructural one due to the way the brain inappropriately reacted to the first injury.

2. We are the sum of our actual physical illness or structural injury + the way we consciously respond to the injury + the way we subconsciously or instinctively react to the injury.

3. This means that injuries due to illnesses, physical causes, and emotional trauma are composed of a percentage due to both structural injury and nonstructural brain injury.

**A placebo cannot treat or improve actual symptoms due to a structural illness or injury. Placebos attempt to treat the nonstructural brain injury that has occurred, which is the way that the subconscious brain has abnormally reacted to produce the symptoms the patient suffers from.**

These symptoms result from an injured subconscious brain that is continually and instinctively reacting. It is these continuous and instinctual reactions that the placebo targets. Let us now explore how the placebo accomplishes this.

Our brain starts out reacting and instinctually responding to the world around us in a way that benefits us. When an illness, physical trauma, and emotional dysfunction occurs, it tests our brain's ability to overcome this challenge by maintaining control and responding correctly. When the brain is unable to respond correctly, the brain incurs injury as well. As a direct result of this injury, it reacts to the challenge the best that it can by creating an improper instinctual memory or response to address the challenge. Once an improper instinctual response or memory is formed, it will become the automatic default method of responding. The result is that these nonbeneficial instinctual memories will always be present. The brain will now be constantly responding even if the challenge it is responding to is no longer present. The effects of this constant responding are the symptoms that the patient experiences.

**The placebo effect consists of the words that are used and the expectation that is raised that enables the subconscious brain to regain control so that it can break the cycle of instinctually responding in a way that does not benefit a person.**

In order to understand how the placebo process works, we have to remember what is occurring prior to individuals taking the placebo. The first thing that is frequently present is a person who is tired of suffering and desires to get better. These individuals attempt to do so by visiting their doctor or making the effort to sign up for the study. These individuals understand through their symptoms that something is broken and needs to be fixed. Most of these individuals have already seen several specialists and have been unsuccessful in trying all the available treatments. Their caregivers have counseled them that there is a new study taking place where a promising new drug is being clinically tested. This drug has been shown to help individuals just like them recover from the symptoms that they suffer from. After listening to this presentation, the individuals sign up for the study and receive a placebo instead of the real drug.

What occurred was that an individual exhibited symptoms pointing to a medical condition. This medical condition was made up of a percentage of actual structural injury and a percentage of nonstructural brain injury. The individual is seeking treatment because he is unable to get better. So there is a desire and need on the part of the patient to improve. If there is a nonstructural brain injury present, then the patient is stuck instinctively and continuously reacting in a way that produces his symptoms. Something has to change in order to reprogram the subconscious mind to stop instinctually responding in a nonbeneficial way. This occurs when the patient is informed that there is a new drug that can eliminate his symptoms and this medication has been successful with others. The acceptance of this offer creates a unique opportunity for the subconscious mind to regain control.

The greater the need and the greater the perception that the placebo will be effective, the more likely the offer of the placebo will bypass the critical conscious thought process and directly affect the subconscious mind. When the conscious thought process is bypassed, the caregiver can influence the subconscious mind, which is the part of the brain where the injury is occurring.

**The subconscious mind unconsciously deconstructs the offer as such: The medical properties in this pill will allow me to regain control so it is not necessary to instinctively respond in a nonbeneficial way that directly produces my symptoms.**

If the subconscious mind accepts the ability of the "placebo" pill to remove the symptoms, then the subconscious mind is able to regain control and overcome the need to continually and instinctively respond in ways that do not benefit it. When this occurs, the nonbeneficial instinctual reactions responsible for the individual's symptoms vanish.

**Placebos work by allowing the nonstructural brain to regain control when the acceptance of the properties of the placebo are perceived as greater than the need to produce a continuous instinctual response that is nonbeneficial.**

The same is true concerning any therapeutic medication or drug that is treating a condition that stems from an injury to the subconscious thought process. If the subconscious mind accepts the idea of the ability of the drug or medication to remove an individual's symptoms, then the subconscious mind is able to regain control and overcome the need to continually and instinctively respond in ways that do not benefit it. When this happens, the nonbeneficial instinctual reactions responsible for an individual's symptoms are eliminated and only the actual physical or structural causes for the individual's symptoms remain.

**In order for a medication or drug to be therapeutic, it has to be able to demonstrate that it can effectively treat an individual's symptoms that remain <u>after</u> the nonbeneficial instinctual reactions responsible for the individual's symptoms are eliminated. If it cannot do this, then a "therapeutic" medication or drug is simply a more effective placebo.**

**This makes sense especially when we remember that some placebos are more effective than other placebos in treating non-structural brain injury. One way to determine if a medication or treatment is valid and not just a better placebo is to remove the nonstructural component before the research study is initiated.**

**An Example Of A More Appropriate Method Of Research**

Imagine what would happen if a study was redesigned in a significantly different way to highlight how our present method of conducting research may not provide a valid conclusion concerning the effectiveness of the medication or treatment being studied.

In this simplified hypothetical study, the goal would be to determine the effectiveness of a new, promising medication for the treatment of fibromyalgia. This medication has been reported to show a significant reduction in pain and pressure sensations. In this study, 2000 similar individuals who suffered from these symptoms of fibromyalgia would have been recruited. These 2000 individuals would be divided into two groups.

The first group of 1000 similar individuals would have undergone the usual double blinded study protocol in which half received a placebo and half were given the promising new medication. After the study is completed, the following results would be found to have occurred.

Percent of patients that reported a reduction in pain and pressure sensations:

Placebo Group   12%

Treated Group   45%

From these results, it is not hard to determine that this promising new drug did significantly better than just taking the placebo alone. Based on this method of research, it seems reasonable to profitably market this drug because it appears to help remove the symptoms of fibromyalgia. Before we potentially make millions of dollars marketing this drug, perhaps we should look at the second group in this study.

The second group of 1000 similar individuals was first treated to address the component of nonstructural brain injury that may be present and is directly contributing to the pain and pressure sensations resulting from fibromyalgia. After treatment, 500 individuals in this group reported that their symptoms of pain and pressure sensations improved or were not present any more, so they were asked to leave the study. The remaining second group of 500 individuals then underwent the usual double blinded study protocol in which half randomly received a placebo and half randomly received the promising new medication. After the study was completed, the following results were found to have occurred.

Percent of patients that reported a reduction in pain and pressure sensations:

Placebo Group   2%

Treated Group   6%

These results are not what are expected when they are compared to the other group. If the medication was effective, then the treated group should have had a much higher percentage of individuals who reported a reduction in pain and pressure sensations. When the patients that suffer from nonstructural brain injury are eliminated from the study, it appears that the new medication is just a better placebo than the one used in the placebo group. The results in the second group of the study are more valid because they recognize that nonstructural brain injury was potentially present in the individuals who were enrolled in the study.

If these individuals with nonstructural brain injury were allowed to remain in the study, the results that would be obtained would not be valid. This is because the question would remain as to whether the medication was a better placebo or if it actually had beneficial medicinal properties. The appropriate way to set up such a study is to remove those individuals who are suffering from nonstructural brain injury so that the true effectiveness of the medication can be determined. When this is done, a double blind study will compare "something" (the medication) versus "nothing" (the placebo).

When double blind studies are performed, we should be concerned when we find that a significant number of individuals are improving when they are given a placebo. We would expect that when a study compares "something" (the medication) versus "nothing" (the placebo) that the rate of improvement using a placebo would be very close to zero. When we see that individuals are improving using placebos, then we may suspect that nonstructural brain injury is present and may be responsible for the symptoms being treated in the individuals receiving placebo alone as well as the individuals receiving medication. Since the administration of placebos is not a comprehensive way to treat nonstructural brain injury, neuroreactive treatment should be considered to eliminate existing nonstructural brain injury prior to initiating the study.

When neuroreactive treatment is performed to eliminate bias due to nonstructural injury, we will truly be comparing "something" (the medication) with "nothing" (the placebo). Research studies performed in this manner are more likely to determine the true efficacy and effectiveness of a new or existing medication or treatment. When the placebo effect of an actual medication or treatment is eliminated, it may make it more difficult to show that many medications or treatments do indeed provide a significant clinical value. Only those medications or treatments that are able to show statistically significant results will be the ones deemed to be beneficial.

# Anticipated Future Books:

*Upcoming Book Number One:*

## The Brain That Allowed Itself To Consciously Change

Wouldn't it be great if you were able to make decisions that benefit you each time you were challenged to do so? This is possible when your conscious thought process knows exactly how to react and respond to the potential challenges that it faces. This book will unravel how the neuroreactive conscious mind functions. It will also provide you with an easy to understand method of how to retrain the way you react and respond so that you can take control of your life one successful decision at a time.

*Upcoming Book Number Two:*

## The Brain That Learned To Be Very Smart

We have often been told that we only use a small percentage of our brain's potential to learn and become smart. This book will teach you how to learn and think by harnessing the untapped part of the brain that we rarely use. This book outlines the process to teach a child to achieve a photographic memory or genius memory through the ability to bypass the conscious thought process through subconscious and instinctual learning. This form of learning can even be done using simple flash cards. The information presented is the result of my work to teach my child to learn in a different way when he was unable to learn using traditional methods.

*Upcoming Book Number Three:*

## The Autistic Brain That Became Functional

This book offers insight into the Autistic mind's thought process while providing creative practical techniques that will improve your child to make him more functional at home, school, and in public. You can give your child the ability to make further functional progress using your child's neuroreactive subconscious and instinctual thought processes.

# INDEX

**A**
Amnesia 105-107, 153-161
Amputation 93-95
Anesthesia 110-111, 125-134
Anxiety 147-148

**B**
Binge eating 148-150
Blame 148-150

**C**
Chemotherapy Complications 98, 170-171
Chicken Pox 59-60
Confusion Reinjury 79

**D**
Dental Issues 175-180
Diabetes 67-79
Diabetic Neuropathy 40, 67-79
Dry Eyes 64-65
Dry Mouth 64-65
Dry Socket 179
Dysfunctional Relationships 49, 50

**E**
Emotional Issues 135-152
Endometrial Ablation 125-134
Exercise 31-32

**F**
Fatigue 13, 61
Fears 150-152
Fibromyalgia 3, 13, 24, 63-64, 99-100
Fixations 150-152
Forgiveness 148-150

**H**
Hypersensitivity 24, 51, 61, 95-96
Hypochondria 150-152

**I**
Interactive Trauma 135-152
Intimacy 50-51

**K**
Knee Dysfunction 109

**L**
Lameness 13
Legal Implications 181-186
Loss of Movement 51

**M**
Memory Issues 153-159
Molestation 171-174
Multiple Sclerosis 61-62

**N**
Nachman 142-143
Neuralgia 13, 103-105
Night Terrors 93-95
Numbness 24, 51, 71, 77,
    98-99

**P**
Panic Attacks 147-148
Phantom Pain 93-95
Phobias 136
Pins & Needles Sensations 61,
    77, 95-96
Placebos 187-195
Post traumatic Stress 24,
    94-95
Psychogenic 25-26
Psychosomatic 25-26

**R**
Rape 171-174
Reason 91-92
Reinjury 77-78

**Root** Canal 178-180
Rotator Cuff Injury 101-103

**S**
Sclerodactyly 64-65
Sjogren's Syndrome 64-65
Stabbing Pain 95-96
Stroke 5, 7, 13, 24, 81-90
Surgery 109-125

**T**
Tics 146-147
Trigeminal Neuralgia 59-60
Tubal Occlusion 125-126

**U**
Uniform Brain Response 3

**V**
Vertigo 122-124

**W**
Weight Loss 42, 161-174